Coping with Epileps
Young F

Susan Elliot-Wright is a freelance writer and journalist specializing in health and parenting. Since training as a journalist while raising her two children, she has written hundreds of articles for newspapers and magazines, and is the author of four health information books for teenagers, as well as *Coping with Type 2 Diabetes* (2006), *Living with Heart Failure* (2006), *Overcoming Emotional Abuse* (2007) and *Overcoming Insomnia* (2008), all published by Sheldon Press. She has a Master's degree in writing and has recently completed her first novel. She lives in Sheffield with her husband.

Overcoming Common Problems Series

Selected titles

A full list of titles is available from Sheldon Press,
36 Causton Street, London SW1P 4ST and on our website at
www.sheldonpress.co.uk

Body Language: What you need to know
David Cohen

The Chronic Pain Diet Book
Neville Shone

The Complete Carer's Guide
Bridget McCall

The Confidence Book
Gordon Lamont

Coping Successfully with Psoriasis
Christine Craggs-Hinton

Coping Successfully with Varicose Veins
Christine Craggs-Hinton

Coping with Birth Trauma and Postnatal Depression
Lucy Jolin

Coping with Diabetes in Childhood and Adolescence
Dr Philippa Kaye

Coping with Family Stress
Dr Peter Cheevers

Coping with Hay Fever
Christine Craggs-Hinton

Coping with Kidney Disease
Dr Tom Smith

Coping with Polycystic Ovary Syndrome
Christine Craggs-Hinton

Coping with Tinnitus
Christine Craggs-Hinton

Coping with Your Partner's Death: Your bereavement guide
Geoff Billings

Every Woman's Guide to Digestive Health
Jill Eckersley

The Fertility Handbook
Dr Philippa Kaye

The Fibromyalgia Healing Diet
Christine Craggs-Hinton

Free Yourself from Depression
Colin and Margaret Sutherland

Helping Children Cope with Grief
Rosemary Wells

How to Be a Healthy Weight
Philippa Pigache

How to Get the Best from Your Doctor
Dr Tom Smith

The IBS Healing Plan
Theresa Cheung

Living with Birthmarks and Blemishes
Gordon Lamont

Living with Eczema
Jill Eckersley

Living with Schizophrenia
Dr Neel Burton and Dr Phil Davison

Living with a Seriously Ill Child
Dr Jan Aldridge

Osteoporosis: Prevent and treat
Dr Tom Smith

Overcoming Agoraphobia
Melissa Murphy

Overcoming Anorexia
Professor J. Hubert Lacey, Christine Craggs-Hinton and Kate Robinson

Overcoming Hurt
Dr Windy Dryden

Overcoming Insomnia
Susan Elliot-Wright

Overcoming Shyness and Social Anxiety
Ruth Searle

Overcoming Tiredness and Exhaustion
Fiona Marshall

Reducing Your Risk of Cancer
Dr Terry Priestman

Safe Dieting for Teens
Linda Ojeda

Stammering: Advice for all ages
Renée Byrne and Louise Wright

Stress-related Illness
Dr Tim Cantopher

Tranquillizers and Antidepressants: When to start them, how to stop
Professor Malcolm Lader

The Traveller's Good Health Guide
Dr Ted Lankester

Treating Arthritis: More drug-free ways
Margaret Hills

Overcoming Common Problems

Coping with Epilepsy in Children and Young People

SUSAN ELLIOT-WRIGHT

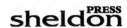

First published in Great Britain in 2009

Sheldon Press
36 Causton Street
London SW1P 4ST

The author and publisher have made every effort to ensure that the
external website and email addresses included in this book are correct and
up to date at the time of going to press. The author and publisher are not
responsible for the content, quality or continuing accessibility of the sites.

British Library Cataloguing-in-Publication Data
A catalogue record for this book is available from the British Library

ISBN 978-0-84709-046-1

1 3 5 7 9 10 8 6 4 2

Typeset by Fakenham Photosetting Ltd, Fakenham, Norfolk
Printed in Great Britain by Ashford Colour Press

Produced on paper from sustainable forests

Contents

Acknowledgements

I would like to thank the many people who so kindly shared with me their experiences of their or their children's epilepsy for this book, and also those individuals and organizations who have answered the numerous questions I had while researching the condition. My special thanks to Roger and Sandie Scrivens for allowing me to include the painful account of the loss of their daughter, Becky. Grateful thanks also to Jane Hanna of Epilepsy Bereaved for her help and feedback on Chapter 2, and to Rona Eade of the National Society for Epilepsy and Dr Pam Crawford for their help and comments on the manuscript.

Introduction

If you're reading this book, it's probably because your child has recently been diagnosed with epilepsy and you're trying to make sense of the diagnosis and what it'll mean for the future, not only for your child, but for the whole family. You may all be in shock at first; you may feel worried, even frightened about what this means, especially if you don't yet know much about epilepsy. Unfortunately, it's sometimes not easy to get all the information you need from healthcare professionals. This may be because not all paediatricians specialize in the condition, or it may just be because there is often so little time available during appointments to ask questions, especially at a busy hospital clinic. This book will hopefully answer at least some of the questions you may have about epilepsy and how it will affect your child.

Epilepsy is a condition where clusters of nerve cells in the brain sometimes 'misfire' and signal abnormally. This disrupts normal brain activity and can cause strange behaviour, sensations or emotions, or sometimes convulsions, muscle spasms and loss of consciousness. These episodes are called seizures, and they can vary enormously in terms of characteristics, duration and severity. Chapter 2 looks more fully at the types of seizure someone with epilepsy might experience. Epilepsy is a tendency to have recurrent seizures, so if your child has only one seizure, doctors will probably prefer to wait and see if another seizure occurs before referring him for testing. Diagnosing epilepsy is a complicated business, because it's not something that can be confirmed or ruled out by a simple test. Doctors will need to ask lots of questions and consider your child's medical history before suggesting various tests, scans or monitoring. Chapter 3 looks at how doctors may arrive at a diagnosis of epilepsy.

The condition is much more common than you might think. In fact, it's the most common serious neurological disorder, affecting between 40 and 50 million people around the world. In the UK, more than 450,000 people have epilepsy – that's 1 in 131. It's roughly twice as common in children as in adults – 700 per 100,000 in children under 16, as opposed to 330 per 100,000 in adults. The good news is that in the vast majority of cases, the seizures can be completely controlled by treatment – Chapters 4 and 5 look at the types of treatment available. It is also fairly common for young people to simply 'grow out' of epilepsy. This will depend on the type of epilepsy your child has (there are many different types), but it is not unusual for someone to have their last ever seizure while in their teens. In a very few cases, people have died as a result of a seizure; this is known as sudden unexplained death in epilepsy (SUDEP) and is extremely rare. Chapter 7 explains the phenomenon and looks at ways of reducing the risk of this happening.

In addition to the various treatments for epilepsy, there are a number of ways in which the risk of seizures can be reduced. This may involve you, or your child if he's old enough, keeping a 'seizure diary' to try and identify potential seizure-triggers. Chapter 6 looks at some of the more common triggers and suggests ways of avoiding them. With young children, it's slightly easier to avoid known triggers – if you know low blood sugar predisposes him to a seizure, you make sure your child eats; if it's tiredness, you put him to bed early. And of course, you'll know that he's taking his medication at the correct time, because you're in charge of the medicine! All this will change as he gets older, and this can be a difficult time.

Chapter 8 looks at ways in which you can help your child to learn to take more responsibility for his condition as he grows up, and also at how to cope with 'letting go' as a parent – not easy when your child has epilepsy. This chapter also touches on how epilepsy might affect the wider family.

Unfortunately, there is still a degree of stigma attached to the condition, although this is nowhere near as bad as it has been in the past. This can make people reluctant to discuss epilepsy, even if they or a member of their family has the condition. But if no one is prepared to talk about it, it's more likely that damaging myths about the condition will persist. A survey carried out by the National Society for Epilepsy (NSE) in 2003 found a number of misconceptions among the general public. One in ten of those surveyed thought that they should put something in the mouth of someone having a seizure 'to stop them from swallowing their tongue'; in fact, this would be dangerous, and could affect the person's breathing or cause them to break teeth. A more recent (2008) NSE survey found that 4 per cent of those surveyed believe epilepsy is contagious, and the same number think it's caused by evil spirits or witchcraft! Chapter 8 also looks at ways of talking about epilepsy and helping others to gain a better understanding. Children themselves want more open discussion about epilepsy, according to research published recently by the charity Epilepsy Action. The research found that while children with epilepsy worried about the stigma, they had a clear understanding of their condition and wanted teachers, classmates and other adults around them to be better informed. The children felt that if adults would listen to their views and discuss the condition openly, they would be better placed to offer support and understanding.

Although the larger part of this book is aimed mainly at parents, I hope that the majority of the information provided will also be accessible and useful to young people with epilepsy. With this in mind, the last three chapters are addressed directly to older children and teenagers. These chapters, while still of interest to parents and carers, aim to reassure the young person, and to provide information and advice that will hopefully help him to deal with the emotional and social impact of the condition as well as the annoying practicalities, such as how to stay as safe as possible if seizures aren't fully controlled.

Epilepsy affects the whole family to an extent, and whether you are the person with the condition, or whether it's your child or your brother or sister, you're probably feeling rather shaken by the diagnosis at the moment. Hopefully, the more you understand about epilepsy and its treatment, the more reassured you'll feel that it doesn't have to impair daily life and limit opportunities. In addition to books like this, there are numerous excellent resources available for people with epilepsy and their families, many of them from epilepsy organizations such as Epilepsy Action and the National Society for Epilepsy (NSE). Resources include factsheets, booklets, information packs, DVDs and videos (see Useful addresses at the end of the book). There is a great deal of information on the internet, much of which is useful and comes from reputable sources. There's also a lot of rubbish, or at least information that's badly written, factually incorrect, or out of date. When using the internet, take care to check the source and if in doubt check with one of the well-known epilepsy organizations. Make use of resources. Read books, ask questions, make a nuisance of yourself if you have to, but get as many facts as you can – knowledge is power!

The majority of young people with epilepsy lead enjoyable and active lives with little or no disruption to their education, often going on to achieve as much or more than their peers, in both their working and their family lives. I hope this book will go some way to helping young people with epilepsy and their families along on the road to a full and happy life.

Note: In order to avoid the rather cumbersome 'him or her' when referring to 'your child', I have alternated between the two throughout the book.

1

Understanding epilepsy

What is epilepsy?

Epilepsy is a tendency to have seizures. It is a neurological condition, which means it occurs in the neurones (nerve cells) of the brain. In order to understand epilepsy, we first need a basic understanding of how the brain works. The brain is made up of millions of neurones, which are linked together like wires or connections in a computer. Neurones are responsible for controlling all bodily functions – hearing, vision, speech, thought and movement, whether the action is voluntary, such as picking a flower or stroking a cat, or whether it's automatic, such as the beating of the heart or the movement of the lungs when we breathe.

Chemicals called neurotransmitters communicate between nerve cells, while electrical impulses travel down neurones. These signals move throughout the brain and into the spinal cord where they can be relayed to various parts of the body to instruct that particular part to blink, breathe, swallow or whatever. There are many different types of neurotransmitter, some of which work to send signals (excitatory neurotransmitters), some to prevent them from being sent (inhibitory neurotransmitters). Most of the time, the action of neurotransmitters is correctly balanced, but like any computer system, the brain can develop a fault, or can be damaged. In epilepsy, the fault occurs when a sudden burst of abnormal electrical activity in the brain causes the normal messages to become jumbled up and sent in the wrong order. This is what causes a seizure.

Anyone's brain can produce a seizure in certain situations

1

– a sudden high temperature, for example, or severe dehydration. Under normal circumstances the brain's controlling mechanisms set a threshold that prevents seizures from happening, but some things, such as brain tumours or infections, drugs or alcohol, can lower that threshold. If something that lowers the seizure threshold is permanently present, seizures will be repeated and the person will be said to have epilepsy.

What causes epilepsy?

In six out of ten cases, epilepsy is 'idiopathic', which means the cause is uncertain but may be genetic or inherited (see pp. 3–4). However, we know epilepsy can be caused by damage to the brain as a result of injury, for example as a result of a road or sporting accident, by an infection, such as meningitis or encephalitis, or by certain inherited conditions or chromosomal mutation. Damage may also occur during a baby's development in the womb, or if he or she suffers oxygen deprivation at birth. Epilepsy caused in these ways is known as 'symptomatic' or 'secondary' epilepsy. Damage to the brain before or during birth may also cause a learning disability, which may be mild, moderate or severe and include sensory, physical or mental health problems. The damage that causes a learning disability may also cause epilepsy.

Who is most likely to develop the condition?

Epilepsy is not, as some people think, linked to intelligence. It can occur in people with average, above average or below average intelligence. However, it is more common in people who have learning difficulties and people whose brains have been damaged or have not developed properly. Although it is also quite common in people over 65, epilepsy is most likely to develop in children or younger teenagers. At any one time, around one in 242 children and young people under the age of 18 has epilepsy, and a quarter of all those newly diagnosed are under the age of 20. However, around a third of young people who develop the condition before they're 16 will 'grow out' of it by the time they reach adulthood. The age at which they have their last seizure will, like most aspects of epilepsy, vary from person to person.

Can epilepsy be inherited?

There are many types of epilepsy, and given that the cause is unknown in more than half of all cases it is difficult to be certain when a predisposition to epilepsy is inherited. Research suggests that some types of epilepsy may have a genetic basis. Genes are the parts of a human cell that determine the characteristics that are passed down from parent to child, such as curly hair, or an artistic talent. So if your genetic make-up can predispose you to epilepsy, then it is reasonable to assume that the predisposition can be inherited. Research is continuing, but scientists believe that a combination of a number of subtle differences in our DNA – our genetic 'code' – may contribute to the development of certain conditions, including epilepsy, and may even influence their response to treatment.

Everyone has their own 'seizure threshold', and this can be inherited in the same way as other characteristics. If a child inherits a low seizure threshold from her parents, something that would trigger a seizure in her might not be enough to trigger a seizure in someone with a higher threshold. It should be remembered, however, that even children who inherit a low seizure threshold won't necessarily develop epilepsy.

We do know that there are some types of epilepsy where a family history has been identified, such as childhood absence epilepsy and juvenile myoclonic epilepsy.

However, if you have or had one of these types of epilepsy,

it doesn't mean that you will necessarily pass this on to your children.

What is the risk of inheriting epilepsy?

The risk of a child developing epilepsy is increased if either parent has the condition, but if the father has epilepsy, the child's risk of developing it is the same or only slightly higher than that of other children. However, if it's the mother who has epilepsy, then the risk is significantly higher. Doctors don't yet know why this is the case. The risk is higher in children whose parents have a history of absence seizures than in children of parents with more generalized or partial seizures, and children whose parents' epilepsy started before the age of 20 are at slightly higher risk than children whose parents developed the condition after the age of 20. The risk graded is about 1:10.

Taking into account these factors that can increase risk, rest assured that even if you are in the highest risk categories – for instance, a woman with a history of absence seizures who developed epilepsy before the age of 20 – it's still much more likely that your children won't have seizures. In fact, according to Epilepsy Action, the probability that your child will not develop epilepsy is more than 90 per cent. If you're worried about this, however, you might want to talk it through with a genetic counsellor. Genetic counsellors can tell you about recognized genetic conditions and talk you through the risks and options, as well as offering advice and support. Talk to your doctor or epilepsy specialist about this.

Types of epilepsy and epilepsy syndromes

There are a number of different types of epilepsy that can affect children and young people. A 'syndrome' is defined as a group of symptoms that occur together to form a pattern that doctors can recognize as a medical condition. In diagnosing an epilepsy syndrome, doctors will take into account the type of seizures, age of onset and whether the child is male or female, as well as his or her general development or learning abilities. They will also look at what is known about the possible causes, which fall into three main categories:

- *Idiopathic* – no known cause.
- *Cryptogenic* – a cause is suspected, but can't be found.
- *Symptomatic* – there is a known cause, e.g. a head injury.

In around 60 per cent of cases, the pattern of symptoms and other information will suggest a recognized, named epilepsy syndrome.

Classifying the type of epilepsy your child has makes it easier for doctors to decide on appropriate treatment, and for them to give an opinion on how her condition is likely to progress. There are many different epilepsy syndromes, some more common than others.

Some types of epilepsy common in children and young people
Benign rolandic epilepsy

Also known as benign rolandic epilepsy of childhood (BREC), this is one of the most common childhood epilepsy syndromes, affecting almost one in five of all children with epilepsy. 'Rolandic' refers to the part of the brain in which the seizures begin. The seizures are classified as partial seizures because only one part of the brain, the rolandic area, is involved. This type of epilepsy usually starts between the ages of three and ten, and often stops around puberty. Most young people will have grown out of it by the time they're 18. Children with this type of epilepsy may experience some difficulties with reading and language or with drawing and visuo-spatial skills, but they're usually well otherwise and do not have learning difficulties.

The seizures often start on waking with a tingling, like pins and needles, on one side of the mouth involving the tongue, lips, gum and inner cheek. The seizure may also affect the throat, causing speech to be unclear and producing strange throaty or gurgling noises. These odd noises are often the first indication to parents that something is wrong. The seizure may also cause twitching movements or stiffness on one side of the face that may spread to the arm and/or the leg, usually on the same side of the body. Occasionally both sides of the body are affected, the child loses consciousness, becomes stiff and has jerking movements of the arms and legs, and may also be incontinent. After the seizure is over she may feel sleepy and want to sleep for a few hours.

Panayiotopoulos syndrome

Also known as 'early-onset benign partial epilepsy with occipital paroxysms', this type affects around one in between seven and ten of all children with epilepsy. It seems to affect boys and girls equally and usually starts between the ages of three and five, but it can present in children as young as one or as old as 15. This type of epilepsy does not usually run in families, although this is a fairly newly recognized syndrome and more research is needed.

The main seizure type here is known as 'autonomic', and over two-thirds of these seizures occur during sleep. If the child is awake, there may be a sudden change in behaviour before she becomes pale and experiences nausea, often followed by vomiting. She may sweat or drool and may become unresponsive. Her head may turn and become fixed to one side, possibly for many minutes. The seizure, which may last 20, 30 or even 60 minutes, often ends with jerking movements down one or both sides of the body. Fortunately, these seizures are very infrequent. She may be upset afterwards and want to sleep, but even after a long seizure, she will return to normal fairly quickly.

Benign epilepsy of childhood (BECOP)

This is sometimes called 'late-onset occipital epilepsy' in order to distinguish it from Panayiotopoulos syndrome. BECOP can start at any age from 15 months to 17 years, but usually begins in middle childhood between the ages of seven and 11. About one-third of children with BECOP have a family history of epilepsy, and some have had febrile convulsions (seizures brought on by a sudden rise in temperature) before starting to have BECOP. The seizures usually affect vision, and in around half of those with this type of epilepsy complete or partial visual loss is not uncommon. Headaches, which may occur during or after the seizure, are very common, and some children may experience a sensation of flashing lights. Rarely, the seizures produce visual hallucinations (seeing things that aren't there). There may be jerking of one side of the body and generalized tonic-clonic seizures (see p. 17) may also occur.

Childhood absence epilepsy (CAE)

This type of epilepsy is slightly more common in girls and tends to start between the ages of four and nine. Absence seizures are characterized by a sudden loss of awareness. The child will stop what she is doing and stare blankly into space for between five and 40 seconds, during which time she will be unresponsive to voices or other noise. The 'absence' is sometimes accompanied by repetitive movements of the mouth or eyes, such as flickering eyelids. These movements are called automatisms. The seizure usually ends as suddenly as it started with the child returning to what she was doing. The seizures can occur many times – possibly hundreds – a day, and are more likely to happen when she's bored, inactive, tired or unwell. Children with CAE usually develop normally.

Juvenile myoclonic epilepsy (JME)

Also known as Janz syndrome, this is a fairly common type of epilepsy which can develop at any time between the ages of eight and 26. However, it usually starts in young teenagers between 12 and 16, and is more common in girls than boys. There are three types of seizure associated with this type of epilepsy:

- *Myoclonic seizures.* These seizures often happen just as the child is waking up. The seizures involve sudden jerking of the muscles of the arms, legs, face or of the whole body.
- *Tonic-clonic seizures.* These are also more likely to happen in the morning, within an hour or two of waking, especially if she wakes earlier than usual or went to bed late the night before.
- *Absence seizures.* The absences usually last for between five and 40 seconds. This type of seizure can happen at any time of day, but is more common in the morning.

Lack of sleep is a major trigger for seizures in JME, so young people with this type of epilepsy should try to make sure they get a good night's sleep – not easy when there are exams to be studied for, parties to go to and films to be watched! Those with JME are also likely to be photosensitive (see below), which means their myoclonic or tonic-clonic seizures can be triggered by flickering or flashing lights.

Photosensitive epilepsy (PSE)

Photosensitive epilepsy is not a type of epilepsy, but can occur in any of the primary generalized epilepsies. It is when seizures are triggered by flickering or flashing lights. Certain shapes and patterns may have the same effect, as can sunlight coming through a line of trees or flickering on water. Other triggers for someone with PSE are watching television, playing video games or using other computer graphics, and looking out of the window of a fast-moving train. PSE usually develops between the ages of seven and 19, but it's quite rare and only affects around 5 per cent of all people with epilepsy, so the number of teenagers and young adults affected is actually quite small.

Localization-related epilepsy

Temporal lobe epilepsy (TLE)

This is the term sometimes used to describe simple or complex partial seizures that start in temporal lobes of the brain. It is thought that the most common cause of this type of epilepsy is scarring as a result of injury to the brain, oxygen deprivation, or past infections such as meningitis or encephalitis or prolonged febrile convulsion. It is not uncommon to find small malformations in this part of the brain that may not have been discovered had epilepsy not developed. There is some evidence to suggest that children who have had febrile seizures (see pp. 7 and 21) are more likely to develop temporal lobe epilepsy when they are older, although many children who have had febrile seizures never develop epilepsy.

The temporal lobes are responsible for many functions including registering and retaining information, hearing, smell, speech and the emotions. Because this area involves so many different functions, seizures occurring here can have a range of symptoms, from a sudden feeling of fear or happiness to an unpleasant smell or taste. Chapter 2 looks at the various characteristics of partial seizures in more detail.

Two rarer types of epilepsy

West syndrome (infantile spasms)

This syndrome usually starts in the first year of life. The seizures tend to be brief, and involve a stiffening of the body and limbs, either in a flexion (bending forward) movement or an arching movement. This lasts a few seconds, followed by a pause, and then another spasm. There may be several spasms in a row. West syndrome can cause a baby to become irritable, and may slow or stop her development until the spasms are controlled. This type of epilepsy is very rare, affecting one in every 3,000 children with epilepsy.

Lennox-Gastaut syndrome

Two out of every ten babies with West syndrome will go on to develop Lennox-Gastaut syndrome, which is also quite rare, affecting between one and five in every 100 children with epilepsy. Children with this type of epilepsy can experience many types of seizure (see Chapter 2), including tonic, tonic-clonic, atonic, myoclonic and complex partial. Absence seizures are also common, and these may merge together to form a state called non-convulsive status epilepticus (see p. 20), where the child may drool, be slow or unable to speak, need help with feeding and may be wobbly or floppy. Lennox-Gastaut syndrome is difficult to control and causes moderate to severe learning difficulties, which may be present before the seizures start, or may develop later.

Ruth's son Josh, now eight, was diagnosed with Lennox-Gastaut three years ago.

Up until Josh was about four, his development was perfectly normal. Then one day he had a seizure while in the bath. He didn't convulse or anything, he just slid under the water, and his eyes were rolling. I called an ambulance and we went off to hospital, but because Josh wasn't well and had quite a high temperature when this happened, we assumed it was a febrile convulsion and we weren't unduly worried. Then a few months later he had another seizure. This time there was no sign of any infection, but the general feeling was still 'wait and see'. Then, over the school summer holidays, I noticed odd little things. For example, Josh's head would suddenly drop, or his eyes would roll. I had no idea at the time that any of these could be manifestations of a seizure. These things began to happen more and more frequently, and soon he was just dropping to the floor.

A round of tests began, including a CT scan, an MRI scan and a sleep EEG (see Chapter 3 for more about diagnosing epilepsy). Before long, it was confirmed that Josh had Lennox-Gastaut syndrome. This was indicated by the fact that he was having multiple seizures and that his cognitive ability was declining very rapidly. Also, his EEGs showed a particular pattern associated with Lennox-Gastaut syndrome.

Even though he was on three different drugs by this time, Josh was still having a large number of seizures every day, some of them quite dramatic and easy to spot, others less so. He would have around 300 absences a day, but he'd go into and come out of them quite gradually, unlike a typical absence where the child just suddenly seems to be in a dream. He just didn't seem to be getting any better. We found it very difficult to get enough information from the hospital. Our paediatrician was great, but the paediatric neurologist – supposedly more of an authority on epilepsy – didn't seem to want to answer my questions. All this was made more difficult by the fact that my husband was in denial about how serious Josh's condition was. He was very supportive and we attended all appointments together, but his way of looking at it was 'When will he be better?', while I knew that it was more likely that the condition would get worse rather than better.

Eventually, after a lot of pushing and persuasion on my part, we were referred to a specialist at Great Ormond Street Children's Hospital. He felt it was inappropriate for Josh to be on these three different medications, and although it was quite a radical step, he suggested we stop all three drugs and try a different one. Since then, Josh has improved steadily, surprising the doctors by regaining cognitive functioning to the extent that his reading age is now three years ahead. He still has minor seizures and some problems with motor skills, but I don't think anyone who didn't already know would be able to tell that he has epilepsy.

We're aware that this type of recovery is very unusual with Lennox-Gastaut, but it just goes to show that anything can happen. I'd advise other parents to keep pushing for new referrals (in the most charming way possible) and to try and keep life as normal as you can for your child, even though that can be quite difficult.

For more information on different epilepsy syndromes, contact Epilepsy Action (see p 115).

Is epilepsy a life-threatening condition?

There are a number of deaths each year related to injuries sustained during a seizure (see Chapter 10 for advice on reducing the risk of injury), but for the vast majority of people with epilepsy, the answer to this question is 'no'. However, very rarely, young people with epilepsy do die during or just after a seizure for no apparent reason. This phenomenon is known as sudden unexplained death in epilepsy (SUDEP). Chapter 7 looks in more detail at SUDEP.

2

Types of seizure

The type of seizure your child experiences will depend on which part of her brain is affected. If the seizure happens in one part of the brain only, it's known as a 'partial' or 'focal' seizure. Seizures that affect both halves of the brain are called 'generalized' seizures; seizures that start in one part and then spread to the rest of the brain are known as 'secondary generalized seizures'.

Partial seizures

Partial seizures are where the abnormal activity starts in one lobe of one hemisphere of the brain. Different lobes are linked to different functions, such as memory or movement, so how the seizure manifests will depend on where the abnormal electrical activity takes place. The most common area for partial seizures to start is in the temporal lobes. Partial seizures start from a part of the brain, though they may also spread throughout the whole brain, becoming a secondary generalized seizure. They may be subdivided into *simple* and *complex*.

There are two types of partial seizure: 'simple partial seizures' and 'complex partial seizures'.

Simple partial seizures are where someone stays fully conscious, and aware of her surroundings. She is unable to control what is happening, and can find the seizure upsetting. Depending on which part of the brain is involved (more specific descriptions later in this chapter), symptoms can include strange smells or tastes, déjà vu (the feeling that you've experienced something before), or an unexplained fear. She might also experience sweating, nausea or a sense of tingling and numbness in her face or arm.

A simple partial seizure can sometimes progress to a complex partial seizure or a generalized seizure. In these cases, the simple partial seizure may be referred to as an 'aura' – a warning or signal that another type of seizure is going to happen.

Complex partial seizures are where the person's awareness is affected, to some extent. She may appear dazed or confused and may carry out strange actions, known as automatisms, such as fiddling with clothes or objects, mumbling, making chewing movements, or wandering about as if she were drunk. Sometimes, someone having this type of seizure might act out of character and do very strange things, such as starting to undress or being affectionate to strangers, without being aware of it. She might make simple verbal responses and be able to follow simple commands, and this can give the impression that she is fully aware of what is happening. This is not the case, however, so it's important not to shout or grab hold of her during the seizure as this could be very upsetting or confusing. On the other hand, she may not communicate or respond to other people at all.

Partial seizures in the temporal lobes

The temporal lobes are responsible for, among other things, hearing, speech, memory and the emotions. If a simple partial seizure occurs in the temporal lobes, possible symptoms include:

- Flushing or paling of the skin, sweating, a feeling of the stomach churning.
- Sensory disturbances, such as seeing, hearing, tasting or smelling things that aren't really there.
- Emotional feelings such as fear, happiness, sadness, or a feeling of being detached or cut off from real life.
- Memory flashbacks.
- Déjà vu, or jamais vu – the opposite of déjà vu. Jamais vu means 'never seen' and is where the person is unable to recognize situations that are familiar to them.

If a complex partial seizure occurs in the temporal lobes, the sorts of symptoms to expect include:

• Chewing, swallowing or smacking of the lips.
• Undressing, fumbling with buttons.
• Staggering around and acting confused – may appear drunk!
• Wandering off.

Sometimes the person experiencing this type of seizure does not become fully aware again for several minutes or even hours, and may be unable to remember anything.

Partial seizures in the frontal lobes

Like the temporal lobes, the frontal lobes control many different functions, including conscious thought, motor function, memory, emotion, speech, social behaviour and sexual behaviour. The frontal lobes are also said to be the part of the brain that is responsible for our personality traits. Because of the functions involved here, seizures in the frontal lobes can be quite unusual and dramatic, which can sometimes lead to an incorrect diagnosis of behaviour problems or psychiatric illness. Someone having a frontal lobe seizure may:

• Display body movements such as sudden thrashing of the body.
• Scream or cry out.
• Be unable to control sexual feelings or behaviour.

Other symptoms include:

• Turning the head to one side; arms or hands becoming stiff or thrashing around; cycling movements of the legs; body movements that seem generally complicated or strange.
• A Jacksonian seizure – this is where a series of trembling or jerking movements begins in a finger and then progresses to the whole hand or arm. It's usually quite brief and may leave her with a short period of muscle weakness immediately afterwards.

Partial seizures in the parietal lobes

The parietal lobes are responsible for our bodily sensations. Simple partial seizures in this part of the brain can cause tingling and numbness, especially in the arms or legs, a warm feeling down one side of the body, or strange physical sensations, such as the feeling that an arm or leg is bigger than it really is. This type of seizure is sometimes known as a 'sensory seizure'.

Partial seizures in the occipital lobes

This is the part of the brain that deals with vision, so partial seizures in the occipital lobes affect how we see things. Someone experiencing an occipital lobe seizure may see flashing or coloured lights or balls of light. She might see things that aren't really there, or she might experience a brief loss of vision.

Todd's paralysis

Rarely, someone who has just had a partial seizure may experience a temporary paralysis in the area of the body that was affected by the seizure. This can last anything from a few minutes to several hours.

Coping with partial seizures

Many young people who experience partial seizures find some of these symptoms, especially those involving the emotions and strange sensations such as déjà vu or jamais vu, quite frightening, especially as they can be so difficult to put into words. It can be helpful for young people who experience these sorts of symptoms to know that their parents understand what they're trying to explain, so if you're talking to your child or teenager about these symptoms, make it clear that you've read up on the subject and can understand what she's going through. And if you're a young person who has experienced some of these weird symptoms, shove this book under the nose of the person you're trying to explain it to; you never know – it might help!

Partial seizures and secondarily generalized seizures

A generalized seizure (see below) is one that affects both hemispheres of the brain. When the epileptic activity that occurs in a partial seizure spreads from one hemisphere to both, it is called a 'secondarily generalized seizure'. The partial seizure is usually quite brief and acts as a warning or aura. Most people who experience this tend to find that they have the same sort of warning each time. These warnings can be an indication that a bigger seizure is on the way, so it's worth discussing this with your child so that she's able to recognize an aura. Sometimes the whole thing happens too quickly for any action to be taken, but being aware of any strange feelings or sensations that occur prior to a generalized seizure can allow time for safety precautions, such as getting into a safe place or position before the seizure occurs.

Tonic-clonic seizures

If the seizure starts in one area of the brain and spreads, it can also cause a 'tonic-clonic' seizure (secondary generalized). An EEG can help differentiate between the different types of tonic-clonic seizures. The tonic-clonic seizure is the most common form of generalized seizure (and what most people think of as epilepsy) and used to be called 'grand mal'. There are two phases to this type of seizure: the 'tonic' phase, followed by the 'clonic' phase. In the tonic phase, the person will lose consciousness and fall to the ground as her muscles contract, causing the body to stiffen. The muscles around the ribs contract, forcing air out of the lungs, and this may cause her to let out a cry or grunt.

After the tonic phase, the 'clonic' phase begins. There may be a bluish tinge to the skin around her mouth and under her fingernails. This is called cyanosis and it happens because the breathing becomes irregular, causing there to be less oxygen in the blood, and therefore less oxygen getting to the body's organs, including the skin.

The arms and legs start jerking because the muscles rapidly contract and relax in turn. She may lose control of her bladder, and she may bite her tongue or the inside of her cheeks. This may seem quite alarming, but it is not possible to stop the seizure, and attempts to do so, especially by trying to restrict her movements, could cause her to injure her limbs.

After the seizure is over, the muscles relax and her body will go limp. She will slowly regain consciousness but may be confused and tired. Her breathing and colour will gradually return to normal, although she may have a headache or aching limbs for a while, and may need to sleep. Recovery times vary from person to person. Usually, a tonic-clonic seizure lasts for one to three minutes, but they can last longer. A tonic-clonic seizure that lasts for five minutes is unusual and could indicate the start of a condition called status epilepticus (see p. 20), where a seizure lasts for more than 30 minutes. Status epilepticus is a medical emergency, so the advice is usually to call an ambulance if someone's seizure lasts for five minutes or more if you don't know how long that person's seizures usually last, or if it lasts for two minutes longer than normal for that person.

Some people experience only the tonic phase, when the muscles stiffen, or only the clonic phase, when the limbs convulse.

Atonic seizures

Atonic seizures, also known as 'drop attacks' or akinetic seizures, are less common. The muscles suddenly relax completely, causing a person to fall forward heavily, and putting her at risk of banging her head on the ground or on furniture. This type of seizure is usually very brief, and recovery is normally quick. However, the risk of injury is fairly high, so if your child is prone to this type of seizure, you'll need to make sure she takes extra safety precautions. See Chapter 10 for more about safety.

Myoclonic seizures

The term 'myoclonic' comes from 'myo', meaning muscle, and 'clonus', meaning jerk. Myoclonic seizures often happen within a short time of waking up and consist of brief forceful jerks of the muscles in one or both arms, or of the whole body. They may sometimes cause the head to jerk or nod. The person is not usually conscious during the seizure, but may appear so because this type of seizure is so brief, lasting only a fraction of a second. Myoclonic seizures may occur several times a day, and can sometimes occur immediately before other types of generalized seizure.

Absence seizures

Absence seizures used to be called 'petit mal' and are most common in children and teenagers, especially girls. They are literally a brief absence of awareness. The person usually stops what she is doing, blinks or looks vague for a few seconds, then carries on as normal. If she is walking or moving at the time, she may continue to do so. The seizure often lasts for only a few seconds, and an onlooker may either not even notice it or just think that she is daydreaming. Because most of us daydream at some point, especially when we're in our teens, these absences can be difficult to spot. Some young people have so many unnoticed absences in a day that they miss out on small amounts of information, which can impact on their learning, and on their social activities and relationships with family and friends. If young people frequently have this type of seizure without it being spotted, parents and teachers may misinterpret what is happening as bad behaviour or rudeness.

Nocturnal seizures

These are seizures that only occur during sleep, but although nocturnal means 'night-time', these seizures can happen at any time when the person is sleeping. Some people have seizures only while they're asleep, which can make diagnosis more difficult and may involve an overnight stay in hospital to allow tests to be carried out while they're asleep. One positive side to this is that many of the problems that face other people with epilepsy will not affect those who only have seizures during sleep.

Status epilepticus

Usually, each seizure a person has lasts for roughly the same length of time for them – anything from a few seconds to a few minutes – after which it stops of its own accord, with no medical intervention. However, sometimes a seizure does not stop on its own, and may last as long as 30 minutes or more. The name for this sort of prolonged seizure, or for a number of seizures occurring in succession for 30 minutes or more without a break, is status epilepticus, which is Latin for 'state of epilepsy'. Status epilepticus can happen in any type of seizure whether convulsive (tonic-clonic seizures) or non-convulsive (partial seizures and absences). A seizure that hasn't stopped after five minutes is considered a medical emergency, whether convulsive or non-convulsive. This is because a non-convulsive seizure can become convulsive, and during a prolonged convulsive seizure, the body has difficulty circulating oxygen efficiently, which means the oxygen supply to the brain may be reduced. Over time, this can lead to brain damage. If you suspect your child is going into status epilepticus, call an ambulance.

Doctors can treat status epilepticus by giving an injection of diazepam or other drug to halt the seizure. It may also be possible for a trained person to administer the drug rectally (that is, via the anus), although they would need consent, either from a parent or legal guardian, or from the person with epilepsy. Some epilepsy clinics now use another drug, midazolam, which can be administered through the nose or inside the cheek. It's not currently licensed in the UK as an epilepsy treatment, but doctors can prescribe it in some cases.

When someone is experiencing a prolonged seizure the aim is to treat that person before a convulsive seizure has lasted for 20 minutes.

Febrile convulsions

This type of seizure may happen when a child has a sudden high temperature. They're more common in the under-fives, and although they may occur more than once, they only occur when the child has a high fever. Febrile convulsions are not epilepsy, but they are worth mentioning here because a child who has had febrile convulsions is at slightly higher risk of developing epilepsy later on.

When your child has a seizure

It can be frightening to watch anyone having a seizure, especially if you haven't seen it happen before, but when the person having the seizure is your own child, it's even more difficult. Hopefully, by reading about the different types of seizure and understanding exactly how they affect the person having them, you'll be reassured that even though your child may appear to be in extreme distress, she probably isn't!

Most seizures happen without warning, last for a relatively short time and stop without any medical intervention. She will not feel any pain, and will usually be fine afterwards, although she may need a short rest or sleep. She probably won't remember anything about the seizure.

Rachel's daughter, Amber, now 13, was 11 when she had her first seizure. Rachel tells what happened:

It was the most terrifying thing to witness. I was ironing in the lounge and Amber had just gone into the kitchen – she'd said she felt a bit sick, so I suggested she have a glass of water then go and get ready for bed. I heard her running the tap, then I heard the glass drop, followed by a thud. I rushed into the kitchen and Amber was on the floor. There was water everywhere and Amber was lying on her back, with her legs and body shaking like mad. Her eyes seemed to be rolling and she was dribbling. I tried to cradle her head to stop it hitting the hard floor but I was really scared I might be doing the wrong thing. I knew she was having some sort of seizure, and I realized I had absolutely no idea what to do. I just sat there, holding her head and wishing my husband was there (he was away on a training course at the time). At last the shaking and jerking began to slow down, and her eyes stopped rolling and started to focus. She looked dazed, as though she'd been woken up in the middle of the night, and she asked me what was wrong – I was crying out of sheer terror! It must have only lasted for a couple of minutes, though it seemed to go on for ever.

Amber was fine soon after the seizure, although she had a bad headache. It was only after she'd started to come out of it that I thought to call an ambulance – I didn't want to leave her alone, even for a second. The doctor who saw her mentioned epilepsy straight away, although it was another few weeks before we had a firm diagnosis of juvenile myoclonic epilepsy, and by that time she'd had another two seizures. It took a while to get Amber's seizures under control – the first drug she tried made her feel worse than the seizures did, so she really didn't want to take it. She'd started to have seizures a couple of times a week, and I was worried about what would happen if she didn't take her medicine. At first the paediatrician wanted us to stick with the medicine, but Amber was so tired and wiped out while she was taking it that she could barely cope with school. Eventually, they agreed to try a different drug, which seemed to suit her better and almost stopped her seizures completely. These days, she has seizures only rarely – the last one was about four months ago and that was when she was very tired. I still find Amber's seizures distressing – more than she does herself – but on the few occasions when she still has them, I don't panic. I know what they are, and I know she'll be fine afterwards.

How you can help

If your child hasn't had a seizure before, or if the seizure lasts for more than two minutes longer than normal for her (or five minutes if you're not sure how long her seizures usually last), you should call an ambulance. What you can do to help depends on the type of seizure.

Tonic-clonic seizures

Someone having this type of seizure may suddenly go stiff, fall over, make jerking movements, cry out or drool. She may also lose control of her bladder or bowels. In the vast majority of cases, she'll recover soon after the seizure and won't normally need medical help. If your child has this type of seizure:

- Don't panic!
- Loosen any tight clothing around her neck.
- Notice the time the seizure starts – if it lasts longer than a few minutes you might need to get medical help.
- Move any hard objects such as furniture out of the way. If possible, put something soft, such as a cushion, pillow or even a rolled-up coat, under her head, especially if she's lying on a hard surface.
- When the convulsions have stopped, put her into the recovery position (see below). This helps her to breathe properly again. Stay with her until she's recovered fully.
- Check for any injuries and seek medical advice if necessary.

How to put someone into the recovery position

1 With the person lying on their back, put the right hand next to the head – like a policeman stopping traffic.
2 Lay the left arm across the chest so that the back of the left hand rests against the right cheek.
3 Hold the left hand in place and lift up the left knee.
4 Roll the person on to their right side by gently pushing down on the left knee.

What not to do

If your child is having a tonic-clonic seizure:

- Don't try to move her – unless she's in a dangerous place, for example, on a staircase or escalator, or in the road.
- Don't try to stop the jerking movements – doing so could cause injury, both to yourself and to your child.
- Don't put anything in her mouth or force anything between her teeth – doing so could choke her or damage her teeth, and it's not necessary – she won't swallow her tongue!
- Don't try to bring her round while she's having a seizure.
- Don't give her anything to eat or drink until she's fully recovered.

Simple partial seizure

A young person having this type of seizure is aware of what's happening, and this can be upsetting for her, so it's a good idea to talk reassuringly to her while the seizure is happening. Remember that a seizure can start as a simple partial seizure but may become complex partial or generalized, so it's worth familiarizing yourself with what to do if this happens.

Complex partial seizure

Someone having a complex partial seizure may seem confused, wander around as if dazed or drunk, and may not seem aware of what's happening. Try to guide her away from danger, such as a busy road or staircase, and talk gently and reassuringly.

Tonic and atonic seizures

The person usually falls to the ground but then recovers quickly. Check for any injuries, such as cuts or bruises to the head, and seek medical attention if necessary. Stay with her until she is fully recovered.

Absence seizures

These are characterized by brief interruptions of awareness, as if she is daydreaming. The seizure often lasts only seconds, but can last longer and could be dangerous depending on the situation she's in at the time – for example, crossing a busy road or frying chips. Try to be aware of the signs so that you can spot an absence seizure quickly, then guide her away from any danger.

When a baby has a seizure

Seizures in babies can be more difficult to recognize than those in older children and teenagers, especially if the baby is very young. More noticeable signs include bicycling movements of the limbs, jerks or stiffening of the limbs or body, or a change in skin colour. Less obvious signs are changes in breathing, and movements of the lips or eyelids. If you suspect your baby is having a seizure:

- Loosen any tight clothing.
- Move things away from her to avoid injury.
- Turn her gently on to her side.
- If the seizure lasts for more than five minutes, or if it's her first seizure, call an ambulance.

After a seizure

After a seizure, some young people need to rest or sleep for a few hours to recover fully, while others are able to carry on as they did before the seizure. Allow your child to recover in the way that suits her best.

If you are a young person with epilepsy, make sure that you give yourself time to recover and if you sustain any injuries, seek medical advice. If you haven't already told your friends, teachers or colleagues about your epilepsy, you should think about doing so – it can be useful for people around you to be sure of what to do (and what not to do!) if you have a seizure.

3

Is it epilepsy? Different diagnoses

The first two chapters have gone into considerable detail about what epilepsy is and how it might manifest. Sometimes it's fairly clear to doctors that someone has the condition; but it can also be quite difficult to diagnose, because there is no one test that can confirm epilepsy or rule it out. Epilepsy is, as we have seen, a tendency to have recurrent seizures. Given that between 5 and 10 per cent of us will have a single seizure at some point in our lives, doctors cannot diagnose epilepsy after just one seizure. However, they will be keen to know if another seizure occurs, and may then begin arranging tests that could give a clearer indication as to whether it's epilepsy.

Some types of seizure are not epilepsy (although may be mistaken for it at first). They include:

- *Syncope.* This is the medical term for fainting, and happens when the brain doesn't get enough oxygen due to the heart rate slowing down. Fainting may cause the body to jerk slightly, which is why it can be confused with an epileptic seizure.
- *Migraine.* This is a severe headache, often on one side of the head, that can be accompanied by nausea, tingling or numbness and 'visual disturbances', such as bright lights, blurred vision or seeing a 'halo' around objects. These symptoms can be confused with those of a simple partial seizure.
- *Breath-holding attacks.* These are not uncommon in toddlers as part of a temper tantrum. The child holds his breath, turns blue because of the lack of oxygen, then loses consciousness. Breathing restarts naturally when he's unconscious, and

recovery is usually swift. These attacks can be frightening to witness, but he's unlikely to come to any harm and will usually grow out of it by the time he reaches school age.

- *Non-epileptic attack disorder (NEAD)*. This is the term we now use to describe non-epileptic seizures that do not appear to have a physical cause. These attacks are difficult to tell apart from epileptic seizures; they are 'real', but they do not involve changes in brain activity. This type of seizure tends to result from psychological causes such as severe stress or anxiety, but the person has no control over them. They often closely mimic epileptic seizures, and may involve a number of symptoms such as changes in behaviour, partial or complete loss of consciousness, and some movement of a limb or limbs. They may be brief or last for several minutes.

Diagnosing epilepsy

If your child has had a seizure, he'll probably be unable to remember what happened, so it's very useful if you, or another relative or friend who witnessed it, can go with him to the hospital or doctor's appointment. The doctor will ask a lot of questions about the seizure and what happened immediately beforehand. This can help to indicate whether or not it was an epileptic seizure. For example, some types of faint can resemble epilepsy, but when someone is about to faint, they often have blurred vision and feel cold and clammy, whereas epileptic seizures often happen very suddenly and with no warning signs.

If, after taking the details of the seizure and considering your child's medical history, the doctor suspects epilepsy, he or she should make a referral to a specialist. According to guidelines published by the National Institute for Clinical Excellence (NICE), this should be a paediatrician with expertise and training in epilepsy, and you should be offered an appointment within two weeks. If your child's epilepsy is particularly complex or difficult to control, he may be referred to a paediatric neurologist – someone who specializes in conditions that affect a child's brain and nervous system.

What the specialist will need to know

The epilepsy specialist will take a detailed medical history to see whether there are or have been any other conditions, illnesses or injuries that may be relevant. For example, epilepsy can develop after a head injury or an infection in the brain, such as meningitis. This is another reason for a parent to accompany the young person to the appointment – parents can usually provide a fairly detailed medical history, and will remember things the young person may have no recollection of. Next, the specialist will ask your child what he remembers, if anything, about what happened and how he felt before, during and after the seizure. Often the main useful information comes from the person who witnessed the seizure, so even though you'll probably find it distressing to watch your child having a seizure, try to notice as much as you can. It may be an idea to write it down as soon as possible afterwards, because stressful situations – and witnessing your child having a seizure can be very stressful – can affect your memory. It may help to think about the following questions:

- Where was he and what was he doing before the seizure started? Was he sleeping, for example? Or watching television? Dancing?
- What time of day did the seizure occur? For example, late at night when he was tired? Soon after waking in the morning?
- Did his mood appear to change before the seizure? Was he unusually quiet, or anxious, or excited?
- Did he mention feeling unwell? Could he have been tired or hungry?
- Did he mention any unusual sensations such as an odd smell or taste?

- Was there anything else you noticed, or anything he said before the seizure that was unusual?

Questions to consider about the seizure itself:

- What first alerted you to the fact that he was having a seizure?
- Did he fall down, or go stiff or limp?
- Did he lose consciousness?
- Did his arms, legs or other parts of the body twitch or jerk?
- Did he seem blank or vacant and unresponsive?
- Did he seem confused?
- Did he behave oddly, for example, mumbling, wandering around or fiddling with clothing?
- Did he lose control of his bladder or bowels?
- Did he seem to have difficulty breathing, or was his breathing particularly fast or noisy?
- Did his skin become pale or flushed?
- How long did the seizure last?
- How did he feel afterwards? Headache? Needing to sleep? Any muscle weakness?
- How long before he was back to normal?

Even if you think you don't remember much about the seizure, any little thing you're able to tell the specialist may help. If there have been a number of seizures, it's a good idea to keep a written record of what happened each time.

Medical testing for epilepsy

If the specialist makes a clinical diagnosis of epilepsy (a diagnosis based on the medical history together with details about the seizure), he or she will then refer your child for tests to support that diagnosis. Although there is no one definitive test for epilepsy, there are a number of tests that can give a clearer picture of what is causing the seizures, and this will help the specialist come to a conclusion. The following tests may be carried out.

Blood tests

A sample of blood may be tested to check overall health, and to look for other conditions, such as low blood sugar or calcium, that could explain the seizure.

Electroencephalogram (EEG)

An EEG is used to record brain activity and shows up any abnormal patterns. If he's referred for an EEG, it'll usually be carried out at your local hospital at an outpatient's appointment. It takes about an hour and is completely painless. Electrodes are attached to the scalp using a special glue or cap, and then connected up to the EEG machine. The electrodes pick up the tiny electrical signals (brainwaves) that are constantly moving between nerve cells in the brain, and these signals are recorded as a picture – called a 'trace' – which can be displayed on a computer screen and printed out. He'll be asked to lie down and to keep still while the test is carried out, because any body movement will be recorded and may affect the result. They may ask him to open and close his eyes, and to breathe deeply to see whether this causes or increases abnormal brain activity. He may also be asked to look at a flashing light; if this causes epileptic activity in his brain it will be switched off immediately.

After the test is complete, the EEG consultant, called a neurophysiologist, can interpret the result. EEGs carried out in children and younger teenagers can be slightly more difficult to interpret than those in young people over 15. This is because brainwave patterns in this group can vary enormously, which can lead to the over-reporting of abnormal EEGs. By the age of 15, an adult pattern is usually developed, although it is still possible to make mistakes in interpreting the results.

A 'normal' pattern shows slightly wiggly lines in a fairly regular pattern; unusual brainwave patterns, called 'seizure discharges', may look wavy or spiky, and may be irregular in shape. One of the problems with the EEG is that it can only provide information about the brain's electrical activity during the period of recording, so a perfectly normal result does not rule out epilepsy, it simply means that there was no abnormal brain activity when the test was carried out. An EEG can only confirm a diagnosis of epilepsy if a seizure occurs during the test, so it can sometimes be a good idea to do an EEG when there is more chance of a seizure occurring.

If the reading from a routine EEG is normal but doctors still suspect epilepsy, your child may be referred for a further, specialized EEG. It's quite common for someone with suspected epilepsy to have several different EEGs to help doctors gather all the information they need. These may include ambulatory monitoring, videotelemetry, a sleep EEG, or a sleep-deprived EEG.

Ambulatory monitoring

The word 'ambulatory' comes from the Latin *ambulare*, which means 'to walk', so ambulatory monitoring simply means 'monitoring while walking around'. This type of EEG records brainwaves over the space of a few hours or a few days, which means it's more likely to pick up abnormal brain activity than a standard EEG, which only lasts for an hour or so. Electrodes are attached to the scalp and connected to a portable unit worn over the shoulder or around the waist, so the monitoring can continue while he moves around during his normal daily activities, and also at night while he sleeps. The longer the EEG is in place, the more information can be recorded and the more likely it is that abnormalities will be picked up or that a seizure will occur. Brainwaves are recorded continuously on a digital memory card, similar to those used in digital cameras. At the end of the test, the information is downloaded on to a computer ready to be interpreted. In addition to the EEG, you or your child, depending on his age, will be asked to keep a written record of his activities and how he feels during the monitoring period. This will help create a much fuller picture of what is happening.

Sleep EEG

A sleep EEG is usually recommended if seizures occur only while he's asleep. He may need to stay in hospital for the test, or it may be possible to do it at home using ambulatory monitoring. Even if he's had seizures during the day, he might be referred for a sleep EEG if waking EEGs haven't shown any abnormal activity. This is because our brainwave patterns change quite dramatically while we're asleep. Sleep can also make the brainwave patterns between seizures more obvious, and this information can help doctors to make a diagnosis.

Sleep-deprived EEG

Deliberately depriving someone of sleep can also cause changes in brain activity. Sleep-deprived EEGs are often used when doctors suspect epilepsy, but standard EEGs haven't shown anything unusual.

Videotelemetry

This is where a video camera is linked to an EEG machine so that it can record both the electrical activity in his brain and what he's doing at the time. After the test is completed, the EEG and the video evidence are stored on a computer. Both recordings are shown on the same screen so that the electrical evidence (the brain activity) and the clinical evidence (what is actually happening) can be viewed at the same time. Videotelemetry acts as an eyewitness to a seizure, so it can help determine the type of epilepsy. This method also means he can be observed for a longer period of time, often over several days, and is therefore more likely to have a seizure during the monitoring, which will pick up the seizure.

Brain scans

Brain scans are completely painless and can produce detailed images of the brain. They may be carried out to see if the seizures have a physical cause, such as a head injury or other damage to the brain, and will involve one of the following:

CT or CAT (computerized tomography) scan

This is a type of X-ray that looks for any areas of damage to the brain that could explain the seizures. Information from an X-ray is sent to a computer, which then displays the X-ray as a series of pictures of slices of the skull and brain. During a CT scan, he'll need to lie, keeping his head still, in a scanner for a few minutes. This type of scan is gradually being replaced by MRI scanning, which is a more sensitive test and gives clearer pictures.

MRI (magnetic resonance imaging)

This type of scan uses a magnetic field instead of X-rays to give a clear and detailed image of the brain. The downside is that he'll need to lie still inside the scanning machine for around 30 to 60 minutes. He'll be asked to lie on a table, which then slides into the cylinder-shaped scanning machine. The tube is enclosed and some people find lying in a confined space a little unpleasant, especially as the machine is very noisy. If you think this may distress your child, it may be possible for him to be given a mild sedative. Although it can be uncomfortable to have to lie still for so long, MRI scans give a much more detailed image than a CT scan and can detect even very small brain abnormalities. They are especially good for assessing someone's suitability for surgery if drug treatment hasn't worked (see pp. 47 and 49).

Diffusion tensor imaging (DTI)

This is a relatively new experimental technique. The DTI scanner measures the movement of water in the brain to detect where the normal flow of water is disrupted, indicating an underlying abnormality. In some cases, this type of scan has picked up abnormalities that have been previously missed by an MRI scan. At the time of writing there are very few DTI scanners in the UK, and the technique is still being developed.

Reaction to diagnosis

Whether you're a young person who has just been told you have epilepsy, or whether you're the parent of a child who's just been diagnosed, you will probably be going through a difficult time just now, and may feel upset, angry and anxious. Although the diagnosis may be a shock, the positive side of it is that at least you now know what has been causing the seizures, which means it's possible to start treatment.

Before the diagnosis, it is quite likely that you knew very little about the condition. Some doctors are better at explaining things than others, but even if you've been given lots of information, you may not have been able to take it in at the time. If you're feeling in the dark about the condition, this can make you feel vulnerable and add to your anxiety. The key is to learn as much as you can about epilepsy so that, although there is no cure at the present time, you will be able to understand the various aspects of the condition and what can be done to minimize its impact, and to reduce the risk of seizures. The rest of this book looks in detail at how epilepsy can be managed on a daily basis. If you're a young person with epilepsy, Chapters 9, 10 and 11 will be of particular interest, as they look in detail at how epilepsy might affect your own life in terms of education or work, leisure activities and personal relationships.

It can take time to accept the diagnosis. It may help to talk about it to people, such as your family doctor, specialist nurses, counsellors and people on epilepsy helplines (see pp. 115, 116). They will be able to give you details of local self-help groups and websites that have discussion forums. Some of these are aimed specifically at parents, some at young people themselves.

When Joy's son Henry was diagnosed at the age of eight, Joy and her husband Michael found the diagnosis very difficult to come to terms with.

Neither of us knew anything about epilepsy before Henry was diagnosed – apart from awful things we'd seen on television or in old films. We knew very little about what epilepsy was, and even less about what might have caused it. Henry is our only child, and we were both in our forties when he was born, so we wondered if that had something to do with it. The doctors asked us a lot about our medical history, as well as Henry's, and that convinced us all the more that it was our fault. I can remember saying, 'But I didn't smoke while I was pregnant, I don't drink – how can he possibly have epilepsy?' I even wondered if it was because I'd had an epidural during labour.

It took a long time for us to accept that epilepsy can just happen for no apparent reason – it's nobody's 'fault'. Michael's parents, who lived very near us at the time, were even more ignorant about the condition than we were. They thought the doctors were only telling us that to 'spare our feelings'. What made it even worse was that they were so frightened by the thought that Henry might have a seizure while he was with them that they were no longer prepared to have him to stay, or even to babysit if we wanted to go out. It really upset Henry – he couldn't understand why he wasn't sleeping over at Grandma's house any more.

As Michael and I found out more about epilepsy, we tried to pass it on to our friends and family, but we did find some people didn't seem willing to listen, which was quite a shock for us. Fortunately, it didn't take long to get Henry's seizures under control, which made life a lot easier, but those first few months were horrible.

Henry's 12 now, and is a bright, happy and confident child. We were very worried that he'd get bullied when he started secondary school, but that hasn't happened, partly, I think, because Henry has a really positive attitude to his epilepsy. He doesn't have seizures very often now, but one of the first things he did when he started this new school was to tell his classmates about his epilepsy. Apparently he told them that he sometimes goes 'a bit weird' and that he might even 'have one of my freak-out attacks'! He loves to laugh about his epilepsy, and to make other people laugh. Some people find that quite shocking, but it's Henry's way of dealing with it, and we're very proud of him.

Claiming benefits

If your child has been diagnosed with epilepsy, or if you're a young adult with epilepsy, there are a number of benefits you may be able to claim. These include:

- *Free prescriptions.* People who have epilepsy and take anti-epileptic medication are entitled to receive all their prescriptions free of charge. Ask your doctor for a form to claim exemption. If you're under 16 (or under 19 and in full-time education) you are entitled to free prescriptions anyway, so you don't need an exemption certificate.
- *Disabled Person's Railcard.* If you are taking anti-epileptic drugs but you still have seizures, you may be entitled to a Disabled Person's Railcard. Children aged between five and 16 may also be eligible. Although they only need to pay the child's fare, an adult can travel with them at a discounted rate. Contact your local railway station, National Rail or the Epilepsy Helpline (see p. 116).
- *Disability Living Allowance (DLA).* This is paid to children or adults who have care and/or mobility needs. Someone claiming DLA must have needed help for at least three months and be likely to need it for at least another six. It's paid at different rates depending on the level of care required. People claiming this benefit are usually assessed on the basis of, for example, whether they can dress and feed themselves, whether they can use the loo or walk around without help. In someone with epilepsy, the nature and frequency of seizures will be considered, so, for example, someone who has frequent seizures, loses consciousness and needs supervision

to keep them safe during a seizure may be entitled to DLA. On the other hand, someone whose seizures are controlled by medication would be eligible only if there was another qualifying disability.

A number of organizations will be able to provide more information about benefits and eligibility, including the Benefit Enquiry Line for People with Disabilities, Disability Alliance, Cerebra (information about claiming DLA for children) and the Citizens' Advice Bureau (see Useful addresses for contact details).

4

Treatments for epilepsy 1: Drugs

Epilepsy treatment has changed considerably over the centuries. The earliest references to epilepsy date back thousands of years, when ancient people thought that seizures were caused by evil spirits and demon possession. Treatment was spiritual rather than physical, and priests were called in to treat the person with prayers or magic.

In 400 BC, Hippocrates argued that what was by then known as 'the falling sickness' or 'the sacred disease' was not supernatural, but was in fact a dysfunction of the brain. He wrote: 'If you will cut open the head, you will find the brain humid, full of sweat and having a bad smell. And this is the way truly you may see that it is not God that injures the body, but disease.' Recommended treatments around that time included enemas and purges, eating mistletoe, and drinking the blood of fallen gladiators.

By the fifteenth century, the 'evil spirit' theory was again popular, with those affected being burned alive for sorcery. Even in the nineteenth century, by which time it was widely accepted that epilepsy was a brain disorder, strange treatments were common. The poet Tennyson, for example, underwent treatment that involved drinking large amounts of water, walking for long distances in bad weather and being wrapped in sheets and dunked into cold baths. A rather more harsh treatment resulted from the idea that seizures came from the genitals and that masturbation caused epilepsy – circumcision or castration! You'll be relieved to know we're a little more sophisticated today!

Anti-epileptic drugs (AEDs)

We now know that epilepsy can't (yet) be cured. But in the majority of people we can treat the condition so effectively that seizures can be completely controlled. The most common modern treatment for epilepsy is anti-epileptic drugs, sometimes called anti-convulsants. The first effective AED was bromide, which was introduced in the mid 1800s and widely used in Europe and the USA. During the first half of the twentieth century, the main drug treatments were bromide, phenobarbitone and phenytoin, but since the 1960s a greater understanding of the brain's activity has led to the rapid discovery and development of more effective drugs, with fewer side effects. Today, the use of one AED will control seizures completely in around 60–70 per cent of people with epilepsy. In another 10 per cent, a combination of two drugs will work. Of the other 20–30 per cent, some choose not to take medication, others will continue to have seizures despite taking medication, and for some, brain surgery may be an option, although this is suitable for only a small number of people.

Doctors still aren't sure how all AEDs work. The aim is to prevent seizures by controlling the excitability of the brain, but how the drugs achieve this is not fully understood. Nor do we know why some drugs are effective for some people but not for others, or why a particular combination of drugs may work for some people but not for others.

Finding the right AED

If at all possible, doctors will try to find a single drug to control your child's seizures. Treatment with one drug is called monotherapy, and is the preferred option. However, if a suitable single drug cannot be found, doctors will try a combination of two or more; this is called polytherapy. Ideally, she'll see the specialist every six months or so, with back-up in between from your family doctor. However, if there are problems with the medication or it doesn't seem to be working, she may need more frequent hospital appointments until things are properly under control.

There are many different types of AED available, some of which are more effective for certain types of epilepsy. It may be necessary to try several different drugs in order to find the drug or drugs that best control the seizures and cause the fewest or least troublesome side effects. This is why it can take a while to get the treatment right. It takes time for a drug to reach the necessary levels in the bloodstream, but the doctor will usually prescribe a low dose at first and build it up slowly to reduce the risk of side effects. Some young people may experience side effects even at a low dosage, and if this happens your epilepsy specialist may suggest trying a different drug.

Sometimes the very first drug that doctors prescribe is suitable – it controls the seizures and does not cause unpleasant side effects. However, you may find that your child has to try several different drugs or combinations of drugs before she finds a treatment that suits her. The recommended way to change to a different drug is to slowly introduce the new one and, once the correct dosage has been achieved, to gradually reduce the old drug. Although this means she'll have to take two (or more) different drugs for a short time, it is important to make sure there is always enough medication in the body to control the seizures. The whole process can take several months and can be very frustrating, but it's worth sticking with it in order to find the most suitable treatment.

Sometimes seizures can be controlled for a long period but then start again. This may be because the patient is 'non-compliant'; in other words, is not taking the medication properly. Obviously this is less likely to be a problem with a young child, because you'll be able to make sure she takes her medicine, but as she becomes more independent she'll be responsible for her own medication and may forget to take it because she's distracted by other things, such as school and friends. On the other hand, it may be that something else is affecting the epilepsy or the action of the drug, for example, alcohol, or illness or other medication, or it may simply be that the dose needs to be increased.

Taking the medication

AEDs come in varying strengths, but for the drug to work properly it needs to reach a certain level in the body, and to be maintained at that level by taking regular doses. In order to achieve this, some drugs need to be taken three or four times a day, others only once a day. For children under 12, the dose is usually calculated by weight. This is sometimes written as 'mg/kg', which means milligrams of the drug per kilogram of the child's body weight. This means that the dose will need to be increased as your child grows. Most children will have the adult dose by the age of 12.

It's important not to miss a dose as this could trigger a seizure. If she *does* miss a dose, the action you need to take will vary depending on a number of factors, including the type of drug, the dosage, and any other medication she's taking, so it's best to ask your epilepsy nurse or doctor in advance what to do should this happen. Also, make sure you read the patient information leaflet that comes with the prescription. Remembering to take AEDs on time can be difficult for some young people, but there are things that can help, for example pill containers or drug wallets into which you put the right amounts of AEDs to be taken at different times in the day. This can be useful for young people who are out all day at school, college or work. You can buy these inexpensive containers from chemists and the National Society for Epilepsy (see p. 116).

As well as tablets, there are a number of different preparations available to make life easier for children or anyone who finds it difficult to swallow pills. These include crushable or chewable versions of tablets, flavoured liquids, dissolvable tablets or powders, and capsules, which can be opened and the contents emptied into drinks or food. Not all AEDs are available in all these forms, but talk to your doctor or pharmacist about the options.

Side effects

All prescribed medicines must, by law, come with a patient information leaflet that gives information about the drug and how it should be taken. The leaflet also contains a list – often alarmingly long – of the possible side effects. Try not to be too worried by this. Remember, these are *possible* side effects, and in reality most people find they experience very few, if any, and that they are often so mild as to be barely noticeable.

Some of the more common side effects include dizziness, drowsiness, poor concentration, fatigue, headache and upset stomach. Less common are swollen gums, acne, weight gain, hirsutism (hairiness), hair loss, hyperactivity in children, depression or even psychosis, which is a serious mental health problem. These are more common in people who have to take the drugs, especially the older types, for a long time. Older drugs such as phenobarbitone and phenytoin tend to have more side effects than those developed in the last 10 or 20 years, but they are still occasionally used when the newer drugs don't work. Doctors may also try drugs developed in the 1960s and 1970s, such as sodium valproate and carbamazepine, which have fewer side effects than the older drugs, but more than the newer drugs.

Some people don't have side effects at all, and of those who do, the majority notice only minor problems that calm down or disappear after a few weeks of treatment. Many people find that their AEDs make them sleepy at first, for example, but this often passes as their bodies get used to the drug. Side effects are more likely if the drug is started at a high dose, if the dose is increased too quickly, or in people who need to take two or more anti-epileptic drugs at the same time. Some side effects can become a particular problem for teenagers and young adults. For example, AEDs that cause weight gain or acne can affect a young person's self-esteem at a time when she feels her physical appearance is most important. Some AEDs can affect concentration, which can be difficult to cope with if she's studying for exams, or starting her first job. Some AEDs can affect menstruation, and some also affect certain methods of contraception (see Chapter 11).

Talk to your child about possible side effects and how they might affect her. If either of you are worried about side effects, talk to your epilepsy specialist about this – he or she may try reducing the dose or changing the drug. Some people are happy to put up with minor side effects, because they feel this is better than having seizures. Others, especially those who don't have many seizures, find the side effects make them feel worse than the epilepsy does, and so they choose not to take medication. However, make sure your child understands that stopping AEDs could be very dangerous, and is the most common cause of status epilepticus (see p. 20). No one should stop taking AEDs without first checking with the doctor or epilepsy specialist.

Increased risk of suicide

You may have heard about recent research carried out by the US Food and Drug Administration (FDA) that suggests that someone taking AEDs may be at increased risk of suicidal thoughts and behaviours. This sounds quite alarming, but in fact the risk is still very small indeed. The research came from almost 200 studies involving 11 drugs and a total of almost 45,000 patients: 27,863 who were taking AEDs (to treat epilepsy, migraine, bipolar disorder and other conditions), and 16,029 who were taking placebo (dummy) drugs. After analysing the results, the FDA concluded that one in 232 patients taking AEDs was at risk of suicidal behaviour, compared with one in 454 who were taking placebos. While there were four suicides in the AED group, there were none in the placebo group.

The FDA has suggested that anyone already taking or just starting AEDs should be closely monitored for changes in behaviour that could indicate the onset or worsening of depression or suicidal tendencies. This all sounds very worrying, but you should bear in mind that all drugs have side effects, and depression is a fairly common one. Even if someone is depressed – and a young person who's just been diagnosed with epilepsy may well become depressed – it doesn't mean she's likely to try to take her own life. Having said that, if you and your child's doctors are aware of the possible risks, it'll be easier to spot potential problems if they should arise.

Side effects in young children

It can be difficult to recognize side effects in babies and young children because they're too young to explain how they feel. Some children have an allergic reaction in the form of a skin rash, usually in the first few weeks after starting the AED. Tell your epilepsy specialist immediately if this happens. You should also be on the lookout for signs that your child feels unwell, or for changes in her usual behaviour.

Many children do not experience any side effects at all, but if there are changes in behaviour due to the AED, these often disappear after a few weeks. If the AEDs are not actually stopping your child's seizures, changes in behaviour may be due to the seizures rather than the drug. Other possible factors in behaviour changes in a child with epilepsy include:

- The severity of the condition and how it affects her daily life.
- How she feels about having epilepsy.
- How other people feel about and react to her epilepsy.
- Where in the brain the seizures happen.
- Normal part of growing up, and nothing to do with the epilepsy!

When the drugs no longer work

Sometimes AEDs seem to become less effective than they were at first. There can be a number of reasons for this, for example the person may have gained or lost weight, taken up vigorous exercise or experienced difficulty getting adequate sleep. It may also be that the epilepsy itself has begun to change.

If your child's AED doesn't seem to be controlling her seizures as well as it once did, talk to your epilepsy specialist about this.

Make sure you get the right drug

Anti-epileptic drugs, like all drugs, have a generic name (a chemical or scientific name) and a brand or trade name. A drug manufactured by different companies will have more than one brand name, and it is recommended that doctors specify the brand name of the AED on the prescription. This is because research has shown that different brands of the same drug may be absorbed at different rates by the body, which can mean that the level of the drug in the bloodstream is lowered so much that it no longer prevents seizures. A number of people have found that their epilepsy has worsened after they switched to a different brand of the same drug. If for some reason you need to obtain a supply of AEDs while abroad, bear in mind that the same drug can have different brand names in different countries.

Interaction with other medicines

From time to time there will be other health conditions that require treatment. Make sure you tell other doctors, dentists and health workers about your child's epilepsy and how it's being treated so that they can decide on the most appropriate treatment for her other illness or health problem. AEDs can interact with other drugs, even common drugs such as the contraceptive pill, over-the-counter medicines such as painkillers, and herbal medicines. The absorption of any of the AEDs or other drugs may be changed, and their potency reduced or increased. There is also the risk that the combination of drugs may cause side effects. Always check with the pharmacist before using any other drug.

As well as interactions between drugs, some medicines interact with epilepsy itself, making seizures more likely. This has been seen in some antibiotics, some sedating antihistamines, some anti-malaria treatments and most antidepressants. This does not necessarily mean that these medicines should be avoided at all costs, but it does mean you need to take the risks into account. Malaria, for example, is a potentially fatal illness, and depression can be so severe that antidepressants cannot be stopped without serious risk to that person's mental health.

How long will my child be on AEDs?

Sometimes epilepsy just stops of its own accord. It is common, for example, for the condition to disappear by puberty, at around 12 to 14 years old. Doctors call this 'spontaneous remission'. About two-thirds of children who develop epilepsy can stop AEDs before adult life.

It can be difficult to be sure that your child's epilepsy has stopped, and she should not attempt to come off AEDs without specialist advice and supervision. If she hasn't had a seizure for a few years, doctors will take into consideration factors such as the cause of the epilepsy and how long it took to control her seizures in the first place, then they will make a decision about whether AEDs can be gradually withdrawn. Coming off AEDs should be a slow, step-by-step process, with the dose being gradually reduced over a period of three to six months until it can be stopped altogether. Abrupt withdrawal could actually trigger a seizure.

In some cases, seizures will return. This may happen in the first few weeks or months, although it's possible for seizures to return after a year or more. There are some types of epilepsy, such as juvenile myoclonic epilepsy, where seizures are highly likely to return if medication is stopped. The majority of young people with this type of epilepsy will need to take AEDs for life.

If someone has not had a seizure five years after stopping treatment, they are said to be in remission. Studies show that around 60–65 per cent of people are said to be in remission ten years after being diagnosed with epilepsy. If seizures do return, treatment should be resumed.

Other treatments for epilepsy

Although the vast majority of children and young people with epilepsy are treated with AEDs, this is not always the most appropriate or desirable treatment. In some cases AEDs simply don't work, in others it may be that the young person doesn't want to take regular medication for the condition. There are some alternatives to AEDs, although still relatively few, despite the fact that research into epilepsy treatments continues apace. The current options include surgery and diet.

Surgery

Surgery for epilepsy is becoming more successful as techniques continue to advance and an increasing number of surgeons become interested in this type of treatment. See Chapter 5 for more about epilepsy surgery.

Diet

The 'ketogenic' diet was discovered in the 1920s and ever since has been a rather controversial treatment for children with epilepsy that has proved difficult to control. With the advent of anti-convulsant drugs, the diet fell out of fashion, but interest has been revived in recent years and it is again growing in popularity. It is thought to be suitable for children aged between 12 months and 16 years, although it can be used in younger babies provided specialist monitoring is in place.

The diet consists mainly of fat. It is low in carbohydrate and 'adequate' in protein. When the body takes most of its energy from fat rather than carbohydrates, the body starts to make chemicals called ketones (ketosis). In some young people with epilepsy this process helps prevent seizures. It is used in combination with drug therapy in children with severe refractory seizure disorders.

The diet is very strict and needs to be supervised by a hospital dietician and an experienced paediatrician. Because of its very high fat content and very low carbohydrate content, many children find the diet unpalatable, so you'll need to come up with all sorts of tricks to help get your child to eat. The dietician will be able to help with this. Older children and teenagers are likely to be more compliant because they can understand that the diet may help reduce the number of seizures they have. It can take a while to tell whether the diet is working – some children show a response within a week, for others it takes longer.

5

Treatments for epilepsy 2: Surgery

Surgical techniques are advancing all the time. Surgery for epilepsy is becoming more successful and therefore is more readily considered than it has been in the past. Advances in MRI scanning (see p. 33) mean that it's becoming easier to find out exactly where in the brain a problem is occurring, so surgery may become an increasingly popular option in the future.

Some people with epilepsy imagine surgery to be the ideal treatment – the 'cure' that means they will no longer have to take medication to control their seizures. It is true that when surgery is performed, it is successful in the majority of cases, though these are very highly selected. In fact, relatively few people with epilepsy are suitable for this type of surgery. This is because it can only be used in people whose epilepsy is caused by a specific problem in the brain, usually scarring in a temporal lobe. This type of surgery is particularly delicate and, like all operations, carries a certain level of risk. Doctors usually only consider it if all other attempts at controlling seizures have failed, and after taking into account a number of other factors; most importantly, they will need to weigh up the potential benefits of the surgery against the possible risks. For this reason they are only likely to recommend for surgery people whose epilepsy has a significantly negative impact on their daily lives. Surgery is still considered by some to be a 'last resort' treatment, although there is now considerable debate about this, with some experts suggesting that if a person is suitable for surgery then the sooner it is carried out the better. This is a particularly important issue with reference to children and young people, because of the implications of earlier surgery on social development, education, relationships and quality of life in general, as well as seizure control.

Surgery may be offered if:

- Drug treatment has not worked.
- Seizures can be seen to come from one part of the brain.
- The damaged part of the brain can be removed without damaging any other part.
- There are no other medical problems that would affect surgery.

If your child has been recommended for surgery, you should be aware that even after having a lot of tests, the surgeon may decide that the operation is unlikely to work, or would be too risky. In fact, only around half of those recommended for surgery are actually found to be suitable. This can be very disappointing and frustrating if you've built up your hopes that surgery could put an end to seizures, so it's best to think about and discuss this possibility with the whole family before the testing begins.

Assuming you decide to go ahead, the next step is to carry out a number of tests; this is known as a pre-surgical evaluation and may include brain scans, videotelemetry and a very detailed EEG, which may be carried out over several hours or days. The aim is for the surgeon to find out as much about your child's brain and the nature of his epilepsy as possible. It may seem as though tests that were done to diagnose epilepsy are simply being repeated, but some of the tests will be more detailed or extensive than the diagnostic tests, while others are necessary for the surgeon to have the most up-to-date picture of what's happening and to be able to pinpoint exactly which part of the brain is causing the seizures.

Types of surgery

There are a number of different operations that may be performed, depending on the type of epilepsy and what the surgeon hopes to achieve. These include:

- *Selective amygdalo-hippocampectomy.* This is the removal of the two structures in the temporal lobe which are commonly the site of seizure activity. In some cases, only the hippocampus part of the structure needs to be removed.
- *Temporal lobectomy.* This involves removing a larger section of the temporal lobe, usually the right side, because the left side of the temporal lobe is the part that controls speech.
- *Sub-pial resection.* This is where the surgeon makes fine cuts in the motor areas of the brain. No brain tissue is removed.
- *Hemispherectomy.* This is sometimes used to treat children with severe epilepsy which is usually the result of serious damage to one side of the brain. The surgeon removes the damaged side of the brain, or disconnects it from the other side.
- *Corpus callosotomy.* This is mainly used to treat children who have very frequent drop attacks (atonic seizures). The operation involves cutting the fibres that connect the two hemispheres of the brain. No tissue is removed. This can be very successful in stopping the drop attacks, but it doesn't affect other types of seizure.

The gamma knife

Most types of surgery involve cutting into or removing sections of brain tissue that are responsible for causing the seizures. However, new and more sophisticated techniques are being developed all the time. One very promising technique is the gamma knife. Rather than using an actual 'knife', this technique uses gamma radiation to destroy the part of the brain that the surgeon has identified as being the cause of the epilepsy. At the time of writing gamma knife surgery is still in its infancy. It is not routine, and is currently almost exclusively used to treat temporal lobe epilepsy. Some people may be able to get this treatment on the NHS.

There are numerous advantages to gamma knife treatment:

- It destroys the abnormal part of the brain without damaging normal brain tissue or surrounding nerves and blood vessels.
- It is painless and in most cases can be done without a general anaesthetic.
- There is no need for an incision, so there will be no scarring and no risk of infection or haemorrhage. The head does not need to be shaved.
- There is a very short recovery time – in most cases patients can go back to school or work within a day or two.

For more information about gamma knife surgery, contact the Gamma Knife Centre (see p. 115).

Has it worked?

It's quite common to experience seizures in the first week after the operation, but this is due to temporary swelling of the brain and doesn't mean the operation hasn't worked. It can be a while before you know for sure how successful the surgery has been, and some experts suggest that it can take up to two years to feel the full benefit. In some cases, the seizures stop or become much less frequent very soon after the operation, but in others it takes longer. Most doctors will prefer to continue AED treatment for some time after the surgery.

Different types of surgery have different success rates, but the results in the more commonly performed operations are generally good, completely abolishing seizures in around 70 per cent of patients who undergo it. Like all types of surgery there is no guarantee that it will work, and for some young people the result is that their epilepsy remains unchanged; in a small number of cases, the epilepsy actually gets worse.

Life after surgery

One of the more surprising aspects of epilepsy surgery is the difficulty experienced by some young people and their parents in coming to terms with the significant life change that comes with being seizure-free after so long. It can be particularly difficult for parents, relatives and friends to get used to a young person's independence, and to learn to 'let go' after perhaps many years of taking extra responsibility for that person. This feeling of things being 'not quite right' will pass soon enough, but it's as well to be aware that it may take some time for the whole family to adjust to a very different kind of life.

Vagus nerve stimulation (VNS)

The vagus nerves are a pair of nerves responsible for carrying information between the brain and other parts of the body. VNS is a fairly new technique involving electrical stimulation of the left vagus nerve via a small pulse-generator (a bit like a heart pacemaker) which is surgically inserted into the chest just under the collarbone. A cable runs from the generator to the left vagus nerve. The generator is programmed to send out bursts of electricity to the nerve, disrupting epileptic activity by blocking the faulty messages that cause seizures. The aim is to reduce the duration, number and severity of the seizures.

It is also possible to generate an extra burst of stimulation by passing a special magnet over the area of the chest where the device is implanted. Your child may be able to do this himself, or it can be done by a parent or other care-giver, either when he senses a seizure coming on or as soon as it begins. This can shorten the seizure, and also reduce the recovery time. The magnet can be worn on a belt on the wrist like a watch.

For some young people VNS is successful in reducing the number of seizures considerably, while in others it may reduce them only slightly. It can take anything from a few months up to two years to tell how well the VNS is working, but the majority of those who undergo the procedure find the frequency of their seizures reduced. In some cases, the frequency of seizures doesn't change but they do become shorter and less severe. For a small number of patients, the procedure brings no improvement.

VNS may be suitable for some children and young people with difficult-to-control epilepsy, and may be an option if drug treatment has failed and brain surgery is not suitable. The procedure doesn't work for everyone, and if after two years there is no improvement at all, the device can be removed.

Side effects

VNS may cause side effects in some people, but these are usually only experienced while the nerve is actually being stimulated. Side effects include discomfort in the throat, a cough, difficulty swallowing and a hoarse voice. They usually reduce over time, but if they are particularly troublesome, talk to your epilepsy specialist to see if the settings can be adjusted.

6

Reducing the risk of seizures

While AEDs are often a very effective treatment, they do not completely eliminate seizures in everyone with epilepsy. There are also some non-medical steps you can take to reduce the risk of seizures. These include learning to identify and avoid triggers, and using complementary therapies.

Complementary therapies

A number of complementary therapies claim to improve seizure control, but there is very little scientific research to back this up at present, although studies are carried out fairly frequently in an attempt to find a safe, effective treatment with no or few side effects. Complementary therapies should not be confused with alternative treatments; 'complementary' means that they should be used alongside conventional treatments such as AEDs, not as an alternative to them.

If you decide to try a complementary therapy, whether it's with the aim of helping to reduce the number of seizures, or to help with another condition, you should always use a qualified practitioner. Make sure you tell the practitioner about the epilepsy and how it's being treated. Contact the Institute for Complementary and Natural Medicine (p. 115) or the British Complementary Medicine Association (see p. 114) for information and advice on how to find a qualified practitioner. Remember to check with your doctor, epilepsy nurse or pharmacist before taking, or giving your child, any other form of medication, including herbal or 'natural' remedies, alongside prescribed anti-epileptic drugs. This is because these medicines may interact with AEDs, making them less effective or causing side effects. Some treatments, for example some Chinese herbal remedies, can actually trigger seizures, so you really need to be ultra careful.

Complementary therapies may improve general well-being and relaxation, and this can be useful. Many people with epilepsy find that they have more seizures when they are stressed, so learning to relax can really help. The most useful types of complementary therapies seem to be those that relieve stress and promote relaxation.

Acupuncture and acupressure

Acupuncture is a system of traditional Chinese medicine that aims to stimulate the body's own healing responses by the insertion of fine needles at particular points around the body. The idea is that our health is dependent on the body's natural energy – known as 'qi' or 'chi' – moving in a balanced way along meridians or channels beneath the skin. The flow of qi can be disturbed by physical, mental or emotional factors; by inserting fine needles into the channels of energy, an acupuncturist can restore the balance. The needles are so fine that most people find them barely noticeable, but if a child or young person is worried about this, acupressure can be used instead. This is where the therapist uses finger or hand pressure instead of needles.

There is anecdotal evidence to suggest that these treatments may be effective in reducing seizures, and this is being researched, but there is currently insufficient evidence that they are effective and safe for treating people with epilepsy.

Aromatherapy

This is where aromatic essential oils are used to treat certain conditions. The essential oil is diluted in a base or carrier oil, and then used as a massage or bath oil. Sometimes the oils are inhaled, or added to water and heated in an oil burner. Some people who experience a warning or aura before their seizures have found that smelling a particular oil, such as lavender, camomile, bergamot or ylang ylang, as soon as they feel the aura can prevent the seizure from happening. Some people say that the oils help them to relax and that simply being more relaxed can reduce the number of seizures. Unfortunately there are still no scientific trials that can confirm this, but in most cases aromatherapy is a safe and pleasant way to relax for both children and adults. It is always best to check with a qualified aromatherapist before using any aromatherapy oil. Some oils can stimulate the brain, which could trigger seizures in some people with epilepsy. These include rosemary, sweet fennel, sage and hyssop.

Herbal medicine

Herbal medicine uses plant remedies to restore the body's natural balance and encourage healing. Some herbal remedies have been found to increase the number of seizures in some people. These include kava kava, comfrey and schizandra.

St John's wort

St John's wort is a herbal medicine often used for mild depression. Studies show that it can affect the blood levels of many types of medication, including AEDs. This means that the level of AEDs in the bloodstream can fall, affecting the person's seizure control and increasing the risk of seizures.

Homeopathy

Homeopathy is a complementary medicine based on the idea that a substance that produces symptoms similar to those present in a disorder can be used, in greatly diluted form, to treat that disorder. However, experts are divided as to the efficacy of homeopathy, and there is no scientific evidence that it is an effective treatment for epilepsy. If you decide to try homeopathy, make sure you use a qualified and registered homeopath. Contact the Society of Homeopaths (see Useful addresses) to find a practitioner near you.

Biofeedback

This is a technique that may help some older children and young adults whose seizures start with some kind of warning or aura. The idea is that, using an electroencephalogram (EEG), the person can learn to control brain activity by watching it on a computer screen. With practice and support from a trained therapist, the person may be able to limit the duration of a partial seizure and prevent it from spreading to a generalized seizure. Biofeedback training can be effective in some people, but requires a lot of dedication and hard work on the part of both the therapist and the young person with epilepsy. It is also very time-consuming.

Lifestyle changes – keeping a seizure diary

One of the most useful things you can do is to keep a seizure diary to help identify the possible triggers for a seizure. If you're the parent of a young child with epilepsy, you'll need to keep the diary yourself, but older children and teenagers can keep their own record and use it to learn how to avoid the triggers they've identified. A seizure diary is also a useful tool for the epilepsy specialist. The sorts of things you need to record include:

- Where did the seizure occur?
- What was your child doing before the seizure started?
- At what time of day did the seizure occur?
- Did she feel unwell or strange before the seizure?
- What was her emotional state before the seizure? For example, upset, angry, stressed, anxious, or excited?
- Was she tired or hungry?
- Had she just eaten or drunk something? What was it and when did she consume it?
- Had she missed or been late with a dose of her AEDs?

These are just a few ideas – note down anything that may be relevant. After keeping the diary for a while, you will be able to tell if there's a pattern emerging: for example, whether seizures are more likely at the end of the day, or whether watching television triggers a seizure. Some fairly common triggers are listed below. Clearly some of these will not apply to younger children, but many of them will be relevant to teens and young adults.

Menstruation

Some girls and women find that seizures are more likely or more frequent just before or during their period. If this happens, mention it to your epilepsy specialist – it may be possible to increase the dosage of AEDs in the week leading up to menstruation, or use a supplementary drug such as clobazam, but this should be done only under medical supervision.

Stress

Everyone experiences stress at some point and it's not always a bad thing – going on holiday can be stressful – but negative stress, for example worrying about exams, or boyfriend/girl-friend problems, can trigger a seizure. If you think your child might be stressed, try and help her learn how to cope with her anger or frustration. The best way to do this is to discuss the problem with her, explain that we all suffer fears and setbacks now and again but that it's easier to cope if you're more relaxed. Learning how to relax properly can be difficult for anyone. See the first part of this chapter for complementary therapies that may help relaxation.

Relaxing

The brain is more susceptible to seizures during sleep and when relaxing. Make sure your child is engaged and involved with enough activities. Taking up a new interest or hobby can help – if she's mentally active and enjoying what she's doing, she's less likely to have a seizure. If she gets bored during school holidays, find out whether there are any clubs, sports or other activities she could get involved in. She could also join a group through an epilepsy charity, so that she could meet and make friends with people in a similar situation.

Hunger

Some people with epilepsy report having seizures when they are hungry. Doctors aren't really sure why this happens, although skipping meals and an unbalanced diet can lead to low sugar levels in the blood and this may be a trigger. Eating regular meals during the day does seem to help people with epilepsy to have fewer seizures. If your child tends to skip meals or just grabs a last-minute snack while running for the bus, try and encourage her to plan her day and meals a little better so that, even if she's in a hurry, she'll always have a healthy snack she can take out with her – something like a few oatcakes and a little cheese is ideal.

Other triggers

Other triggers include alcohol and other recreational drugs (see p. 105) and flashing lights (see p. 97).

7

Sudden unexpected death in epilepsy (SUDEP)

SUDEP, where someone dies during or just after a seizure for no apparent reason – where there is no obvious injury, for example – is a phenomenon that can occasionally occur in young people with epilepsy. It's rare in children under 16, and although there has been little research on this, the research currently available suggests that when it does occur in children it is more common in those who have other difficulties as well, such as difficult-to-control seizures, or learning or other disabilities. We don't know exactly how many deaths are as a result of SUDEP, but it is thought to be around one in every 1,000 people with epilepsy – about the same risk as smoking ten cigarettes a day. For people with severe epilepsy, the risk increases to between one in 100 and one in 300, and it's around one in 50 for those who have been referred for epilepsy surgery but considered unsuitable. In the UK, around 500 people a year die from SUDEP.

Doctors have known about SUDEP for a very long time, but it seems to be poorly understood and something of a taboo subject. Many people with epilepsy say that their doctors have never even mentioned SUDEP, and that they have received no information about the phenomenon. National guidelines for clinicians recommend that patients and their families are given information on SUDEP, but some doctors argue that they don't want to alarm patients and their families unnecessarily, and it's certainly true that SUDEP is rare. However, many patient organizations and families who have lost a child, sibling or friend to SUDEP believe this to be rather skewed logic. If people with epilepsy are not told about the risks, they argue, how can they possibly reduce those risks? Some organizations argue that a substantial proportion of epilepsy deaths could have been prevented if the person had been better informed.

SUDEP is an area in which there is still little research. One of the problems is that in many cases the person dies alone, at night, which often means there are no witnesses. This clearly makes it difficult to establish the cause of death. It is thought that a seizure might interfere with areas of the brain that control breathing or the heart. It's not particularly uncommon for someone to stop breathing during a seizure, but in most cases he would start to breathe again when the seizure was over. In those who have died from SUDEP, it is clear that breathing did not start again after the seizure. In most of these cases, doctors aren't sure whether there was already a weakness in that person's heart or lungs, or whether the death was due entirely to the epilepsy. Where the heart is concerned, it is thought that the abnormal electrical discharges that cause a seizure may also affect the heart's rhythm, causing it to beat abnormally fast. This can lead to a condition called ventricular fibrillation, where the heart muscles become weak and start to contract randomly and ineffectively. The heart is no longer able to pump blood around the body, and if the condition isn't treated immediately death follows quickly.

SUDEP is most likely to occur in young adults between the ages of 20 and 30, although it can sometimes occur in younger or older people. In most cases, then, the person who dies is young, and apparently fit and healthy. It seems to affect more males than females.

SUDEP is rare, but some people appear to be slightly more at risk than others. Particular risk factors include:

- Generalized tonic-clonic seizures.
- Seizures that are not adequately controlled.

- Seizures during sleep.
- Not taking prescribed anti-epileptic medication.
- Frequent or sudden changes to anti-epileptic medication.
- Living alone (so seizures are unwitnessed).
- Drinking too much alcohol.

Reducing the risk of SUDEP

If you are the parent or carer of a young person with epilepsy, you may be able to help reduce the risk of SUDEP.

Many SUDEP deaths occur when the person is alone (though this isn't always the case). If you happen to be with the young person when he has a seizure, it's a good idea to stay with him for 15–20 minutes after the seizure has ended, just to make sure he's back to normal.

Remember, it's not uncommon for someone to stop breathing during a seizure, and breathing usually restarts on its own. However, in a few rare cases, as we've seen, breathing doesn't restart spontaneously. If breathing hasn't restarted after a seizure, try moving him, or even just moving his limbs – this may help to get him breathing again. If he's had a tonic-clonic seizure, roll him on to his side and put him in the recovery position (see p. 23).

There are a number of 'seizure alert devices' available that can detect changes that may indicate a seizure and set off an alarm to alert the parent or carer. The devices vary in terms of what they can detect and their effectiveness, but the range includes detecting changes or interruptions in breathing, changes in heart rate or body temperature, and unusual or violent movements. Devices work by means of a sensor, which is fitted under the mattress. When a seizure is detected, a loud alarm will sound so that you can get to the child quickly and take the appropriate action.

These devices may be recommended for children who have nocturnal seizures, but it should be borne in mind that the current evidence base for their effectiveness is weak, so there is a slight danger of a 'false sense of security'. Contact one of the epilepsy helplines (see Useful addresses) for details of companies that supply the alarms. In cases of financial difficulty, it may be possible for some families to receive funding for a bed alarm. Contact the Muir Maxwell Trust at <www.muirmaxwelltrust.com>.

If you are a young person with epilepsy, there is a great deal you can do to reduce your risk of SUDEP.

- Make sure your seizures are as well controlled as they can possibly be. If your current medication does not control your seizures adequately, ask to be referred to an epilepsy specialist. There may be other treatment options (see Chapter 4) that you could discuss at this point.
- Make sure you take your prescribed medication, even if you have to set all sorts of electronic reminders!
- Avoid activities or situations that may trigger seizures (see Chapter 6).
- Make sure you don't run out of your medication – this is more likely to happen at weekends or bank holidays, and if you go away on holiday.
- Never change the dose or stop your medication without checking with your epilepsy specialist.
- Always attend regular appointments to review your treatment in case changes are required – for example, increased body weight may mean you need a different dosage.
- If you have difficult-to-control epilepsy, you may need to be referred to a specialist epilepsy clinic.

Bereavement

If you have lost a child or other person close to you because of SUDEP, you will probably be experiencing a variety of emotions. As well as experiencing the trauma associated with any sudden death of a child or young person, you might feel bewildered by what has happened, or angry that you weren't given information about this possibility. It may help to get in touch with Epilepsy Bereaved (see p. 115 for contact details), a charity set up by bereaved relatives to provide support and information to those bereaved by SUDEP. Epilepsy Bereaved also tries to enable relatives to channel their grief positively in the cause of the charity. Their aims are to dedicate research into the prevention of SUDEP and other epilepsy deaths, to educate and campaign to improve epilepsy services, and to ensure that information on reducing risks of SUDEP is readily available to people with epilepsy and their families.

Roger and Sandie lost their beloved daughter Becky in 2004, just three months short of her twelfth birthday, and just days after she was diagnosed with a form of epilepsy that is known to respond well to medication. SUDEP had never been mentioned to them, and the first time they came across the acronym was three days after Becky's death when they found the Epilepsy Bereaved website. Since their daughter's death, Roger and Sandie have, with the support of Epilepsy Bereaved, worked tirelessly to raise awareness of SUDEP, both among the general public and among healthcare professionals. This is an extract from Becky's story as told by her parents.

> Becky suffered her first ever seizure in September 2001. She was promptly seen by a registrar at the local hospital, but despite all the clues (so obvious in hindsight) we were sent on our way with a 'nothing to worry about, it's probably migraine, we can't do anything more unless the seizures become regular and frequent' message. After a further two years of sporadic night-time fits, those words of comfort converted to concern when seizures appeared during the first weeks of January, February and March 2004. We pushed for a referral to a paediatrician who did think that Becky might be suffering from epileptic seizures in addition to migraine. He arranged for her to undergo EEG and MRI scans. But seizure control medication was 'out of the question for a child of this age' (we have subsequently found this statement to be totally unfounded) and no mention was made of SUDEP. She died three days before we were due to visit the hospital to discuss the MRI results.

Three days after her death we heard about sudden unexpected death in epilepsy for the first time. Even then it was in the form of a passing reference from the Coroner's Office. Then some web searching uncovered the Epilepsy Bereaved site and our first viewing of the acronym SUDEP … and the horror associated with it.

Becky's earlier life had, in hindsight, given clues to her epilepsy. She appeared to have early learning difficulties. Was she a dyslexia sufferer? We investigated but the results seemed to confirm she was actually a very bright girl who often just 'drifted off' for brief periods. These absences were probably early signs of her epilepsy. In fact, during the last months of Becky's life she experienced brief flashing light/bright colour visual disturbances on a daily basis and was concerned that her teachers might think she wasn't concentrating during lessons. These daytime experiences continued to be diagnosed as migraine up until her death.

Becky was a beautiful, fun-loving, intelligent, caring girl who was much loved by all who knew her. She loved to participate and be involved with others and always gave her best at everything she tried – be it work or play! How we miss seeing how she would have developed into adulthood.

Becky's inquest was held some five months after her death. We had no idea what to expect and found the experience very daunting. During the proceedings it became clear that up until that day, the Coroner's knowledge of SUDEP had been extremely limited, to say the least. We are now striving to ensure that Becky's death was not in vain. We are working with the local NHS Trust to improve the system for children with suspected epilepsy; this will be a long and ongoing project. We are also supporting the Education and Awareness project at Epilepsy Bereaved to promote awareness of ways to reduce epilepsy deaths.

Roger and Sandie urge anyone who has children, friends or family who have epilepsy or who have demonstrated symptoms, to visit the Epilepsy Bereaved website at <www.sudep. org>. They say: 'On that site, as well as learning more about this much misunderstood condition, you can read our Becky's story in full.'

8

Helping your child (and the rest of the family) to cope

Living with epilepsy on a daily basis can be difficult for the whole family. The first few weeks after diagnosis will probably be taken up with medical appointments as doctors try to establish an appropriate treatment plan. But when things settle down a bit, you'll start to think about the impact your child's epilepsy might have on his, and your, daily life.

Talking about epilepsy

Sadly, although we understand epilepsy much better than we did in the past, the condition can still carry a stigma. This arises through fear, misunderstanding and ignorance, and can sometimes have more impact on the life of the person with epilepsy than the condition itself does. One of the problems is that because of the possible stigma attached, people with epilepsy (and their families) are often reluctant to talk about it. This means that those around them remain in ignorance and therefore the fear and misunderstanding continues – it's a vicious circle. The same thing applies to many other health conditions as well. For some reason health – or more specifically, ill-health – is a taboo subject. The best way to combat taboos is to smash them. If you're a young person with epilepsy, Chapters 9 and 11 touch on how you might deal with any problems that may arise as a result of this. If it's your child who's just been diagnosed, you're probably feeling apprehensive about telling people, but it's very important to tell anyone who will be caring for your child about his epilepsy. This includes his school or nursery, childminders, babysitters, grandparents and other family members who look after him, and, if he goes to a friend's house to play, the friend's parents.

The information you need to give will depend on how much the person you're telling already knows about epilepsy. Your family and friends, for example, may have very little prior knowledge, whereas teachers might be better informed. Most people will feel much more relaxed once they understand a bit more about the condition, so try to explain as much as you can, and perhaps offer them some basic information leaflets. Close family members might prefer to read a book like this one, or look at the websites of the National Society for Epilepsy (NSE) or Epilepsy Action (see Useful addresses). If your child's school doesn't seem particularly well-informed, talk to the epilepsy organizations just mentioned about what materials they can provide – they may be able to offer helpful leaflets, books or information packs. Also, you may be able to arrange for an epilepsy nurse to visit the school to give a talk to staff and children about what epilepsy is and who it can affect – that is, absolutely anyone!

Even people who know a lot about epilepsy in general will need to know specifically about your child's epilepsy if they're caring for him at any point. You'll need to tell them:

- How many seizures your child tends to have.
- What form the seizures take and how long they last.
- Whether there's anything in particular that might trigger them.
- What first aid might be required.
- Whether your child needs to rest or sleep after the seizure and for how long.
- Whether he gets an aura or warning of a seizure.

- Whether he needs to take any medication (most schools have a policy on prescription drugs).
- What action you would like the person to take in the unlikely event of an emergency.

You'll probably find that once people understand more about the condition they'll be less afraid of it, which will mean *they* are able to talk about it. This has a far-reaching effect in that more people will understand the condition and the taboo will eventually be broken down.

Josh has Lennox-Gastaut syndrome, and at one time his seizures were so violent that there was a very real danger of him being injured during a seizure. His mum Ruth says:

Josh was having very frequent seizures and often he would crash to the floor, convulsing violently. We'd explained his condition to his school, and it wasn't long before he had a special needs statement, which meant he was able to have full-time help and support while at school. This made things a lot easier, but there was still a danger that Josh might suffer a head injury during a seizure, so we thought it best for him to wear a protective helmet. We told the school about this, and the head teacher arranged a special assembly on the Friday to explain to the whole school about Josh's epilepsy, and that when he came to school on Monday he would be wearing a helmet and this was why.

Obviously, wearing the helmet marked Josh out as being different, but by the time the children saw him with it they understood why he was wearing it, and I think this made a difference to their perceptions. The problem is that even though you can explain to the school and to family and friends, you can't explain to everyone in the street, and until we start talking more openly about epilepsy there will be a stigma attached to the condition.

When Josh's specialist at Great Ormond Street suggested we think about the risks of head injury and weigh them up against the risks of Josh suffering as a result of the stigma, we decided to ditch the helmet. It was a slightly scary step to take, but there's a great danger of wrapping children with epilepsy in cotton wool, and in some cases this can adversely affect their lives more than the epilepsy does. (See p. 10 for Ruth's account of Josh's diagnosis and treatment.)

Talking to your child about his epilepsy

Obviously, when and how you talk to your child about his epilepsy will depend on his level of understanding. Epilepsy is a complex condition, and trying to explain it to a young child or a child who also has a learning disability can be difficult, but this should not put you off. Most children will cope much better with the condition if they understand what's happening. It's a good idea to read up on the subject yourself first, so that you will be in a better position to answer your child's questions. If he asks a question you cannot answer, just tell him that you don't know yet, but you'll find out. If your reading material doesn't supply the answer it might be worth trying one of the help-lines (see p. 114); if his question is specific to his own epilepsy you'll need to talk to your epilepsy nurse or doctor. Epilepsy organizations such as Epilepsy Action and the National Society for Epilepsy (NSE) have a range of useful materials, including videos and DVDs, that can help explain epilepsy to younger and older children, to adults, or to people with learning disabilities. Depending on how old/mature your child is, you may decide that the materials aimed at adults are more suitable for him.

Give your child as much or as little information as you feel he's ready for. Don't swamp him with too much, but on the other hand don't skim the important things, like seizure control and staying safe. Try to be as open and honest as you can about the condition. Don't worry too much if he doesn't want to talk about his epilepsy. It's his right not to discuss it if that's how he feels; just make sure he knows he can discuss it if he wants to. You'll need to help him to understand that treating and managing his condition is important, but at the same time you've got to be careful not to overdramatize or overstate the importance.

It's a difficult route to navigate, and dealing with a young person who might be very angry about his condition, not to mention the sheer angst of growing up, can be difficult for parents. Don't feel guilty about being cross with or infuriated by your child – it's normal, especially during the teenage years when parenting becomes notoriously difficult, whether your child has epilepsy or not! Try to remember that you're not the only family going through this. There's plenty of help and support out there from epilepsy organizations, support groups and online forums, both for you as a parent and for your child as a young person learning to live with epilepsy. You can find out about these through epilepsy organizations such as NSE and Epilepsy Action.

Anthony's daughter Sophie was three when she was diagnosed. She's now 13 and things have become a little more difficult in the last few years. Anthony explains:

Thinking back, Sophie probably had epilepsy even as a baby, but she was our first child and we didn't really have anything to compare it with. She was just three when she started to have more obvious seizures. The first time, my wife noticed that Sophie's head was nodding in an odd way. I didn't actually see it, so I didn't perhaps take it as seriously as I could have, but my wife had worked with a family with a child who had epilepsy, so she was more aware. Soon after that we were at the zoo one day when Sophie suddenly screamed and came running over to me. She was nodding her head again, and my wife said, 'That's it, that's what she was doing before!'

We saw our GP who initially brushed the whole thing aside, so we asked to be referred to a paediatrician who very quickly diagnosed epilepsy and got Sophie on to anti-epileptic medication. The daytime seizures disappeared almost completely and now, ten years on, she usually has seizures only at night. Having said that, I'm fairly sure she's still having absences during the day, but they're quite brief so it's difficult to tell. During the night-time seizures, the screams still occur (like that first time, which was very scary), but that's only the seizures that we notice – I wonder whether she may be having silent night-time seizures that we *don't* notice.

Even though things have improved considerably, Sophie has some behaviour problems which we're sure are linked to her epilepsy. She tends to fly off the handle easily, and she feels very angry much of the time, especially if she feels she's not the centre of attention. This all seems to get worse just before a seizure. Sometimes she seems to deliberately wind us up. For example, when my wife reminds her to take her medicine (she needs to take it twice a day) she'll say, 'I don't think I'll bother to take it any more.' Similarly, we have regular counselling with a specially trained counsellor, and sometimes my wife and I see the counsellor, sometimes we see her along with Sophie, and sometimes Sophie sees her alone. Sophie seems to really enjoy the sessions she has on her own with the counsellor, but each time she comes out, she makes it seem like she never wants to do it again!

I know from talking to other people who have epilepsy just how marginalized they feel. That, together with being 13, must be pretty difficult. We know that Sophie's epilepsy may get worse as she enters puberty, and in fact she had quite a big seizure the other day, but in general things have been improving over the last few months. It's a difficult time for the whole family, but we know it could be much worse, and we're working on it.

Siblings

A diagnosis of epilepsy can be difficult for all the family, and in the case of siblings a number of problems may arise as a result of fears that almost certainly develop through ignorance or misunderstanding of the condition. We've already seen how educating and informing people about epilepsy can make them much more relaxed about it; unfortunately, when you're worried about one of your children and you're busy dealing with potential areas of difficulty, such as school and childcare, it's easy to overlook your other children, especially if they're quite young. Try to take some time to discuss the situation as a family, but also create an opportunity for each child to spend time alone with you or the other parent so that he can ask questions or talk about any aspect of his sibling's epilepsy that he finds particularly worrying.

As already mentioned, there are some very good information materials available to suit most age ranges, and these should help you to reassure your child, but he may still worry about specific issues and you'll need to answer each question honestly, but hopefully in such a way that he'll feel happier about the situation. Common worries include:

- Fear that he too may develop epilepsy.
- Fear that his sibling might die.
- Fear that he'll be alone with his sibling during a seizure.
- Fear that his friends will pick on him.
- Fear that you love his sibling more than him.

Obviously, how you reassure your child will depend on a number of factors, including his age and maturity, whether he's younger or older than his sibling, and the type of epilepsy his sibling has. As a rough guide, if he's worried about developing epilepsy himself, explain that although it can happen to anyone, the risk is very small indeed. If he's afraid his sibling might die, you can reassure him that while some deaths do occur as a result of epilepsy, this is extremely rare. If he's afraid of being alone with his sibling when a seizure occurs, make sure he understands what happens during a seizure, and show him what to do, whether it's simply talking to and reassuring his sibling during the seizure, or whether he needs to take any other action (such as phoning an ambulance in an emergency situation – see p. 23). If he's afraid his friends will pick on him, try and encourage him to talk to them about his sibling's epilepsy – it's the same old story: the more that people understand about the condition, the less afraid they'll be, and consequently the less likely they are to be unpleasant or insensitive about it.

Finally, even though he's unlikely to tell you this, it's not unusual for a child to feel that his parents no longer love him as much as the child with epilepsy. This probably arises because he sees you worrying about his sibling, giving him lots of attention, perhaps even being over-concerned and protective. The best way round this is probably to include your other children as much as possible in discussions about the epilepsy, its treatment and how it affects all your lives. Make some 'special time' for each child – time when that child alone has your or your partner's undivided attention. Try to alternate this so that sometimes he has time alone with Mum, sometimes with Dad. This can be a good time to encourage him to tell you about any worries he may have. If possible, try and have this time together when your partner or another responsible person is in the house. That way if a seizure occurs during a sibling's special time, you won't have to abandon him in order to attend to the child with epilepsy, thus helping to maintain a sense of normality for all your children.

Depression

Depression is fairly common among young people, but someone with epilepsy is even more likely to become depressed. We all feel low sometimes, and it's perfectly normal for your child to feel low after being diagnosed with epilepsy. But gradually, as he starts to understand his condition and get his seizures under control, he should start to feel less sad and eventually return to having the odd 'off' times like most young people. However, if his sadness and low mood last for longer than a few days, he may be depressed. Depression affects different people in different ways, but listed below are some of the signs to look out for.

- Persistent low mood, often worse in the mornings.
- Being tearful, feeling bleak and hopeless.
- Being unable to enjoy social or leisure activities.
- Loss of interest in friends and social life.
- Sleep difficulties – being unable to sleep, or sleeping too much.
- Lack of energy, fatigue.
- Slowed thinking, speech and/or movements.
- Being unable to concentrate.

- Anxiety, panic attacks.
- Suicidal thoughts and ideas.

He doesn't need to experience all of these symptoms to be suffering from depression, but by keeping an eye on him over the course of a week or so you'll be able to see whether any of these symptoms are lasting longer than would be considered 'normal'.

Possible causes

Although depression in people with epilepsy can have the same causes as in someone who doesn't have the condition – for example, stress or bereavement – there are some factors specific to epilepsy that could trigger depression.

Diagnosis

It's well known that depression can occur as a result of trauma and distress, and a diagnosis of epilepsy can indeed be traumatic and distressing. In fact, the diagnosis can cause a response similar to that experienced by someone who has been bereaved: disbelief, denial, anger and depression. Your child is facing a life-changing situation at a time when he may just have been beginning to map out his future. Suddenly everything might be different: he may find it more difficult, or even impossible, to follow the career path he'd planned; his activities and hobbies may be affected; he may worry about the effect on his friendships and relationships. In addition, he's having to cope with seizures, regular visits to doctors and hospitals, and the possibility that he may have to take medication for the rest of his life.

In some cases, however, a young person may have been depressed for some time before diagnosis. It's possible that now a diagnosis is in place and treatment can begin the depression may actually begin to lift, once the condition is brought under control.

Medication

Sometimes depression can be a side effect of anti-epileptic medication. The patient information leaflet that comes with the drug may warn of this, but even if it doesn't, it's still possible that the depression may be related to the medication. If you suspect this, discuss the situation with your specialist to see whether it might be appropriate to change the dosage or the drug.

Seizures

We don't know exactly why, but some people have changes in mood in the period before a seizure, and depression may occur as part of an aura or warning before a more obvious seizure occurs. Similarly, a brief period of depression is common following a seizure.

The underlying cause of epilepsy

As we have seen, epilepsy is sometimes caused by damage to the brain. This can occur for many reasons, including head injury, a difficult birth, or an infection such as meningitis or encephalitis. Given that our brains control our moods and emotions, it's not surprising that damage to the brain and the resulting disruption to brain function can also cause depression. Research suggests that depression is more common in people with damage to the frontal and temporal lobes than in those with damage to other parts of the brain. Having said that, there are plenty of people with brain damage who do not suffer from depression.

Treatment for depression

If you suspect your child may be depressed, encourage him to talk about how he's feeling, and to discuss it with the doctor. It's no good telling him to 'cheer up' or 'pull yourself together'. If he has depression, the chemicals in his brain that govern his mood make it impossible for him to 'cheer up'. Depression is a serious condition that requires treatment, possibly with medication, counselling, cognitive behaviour therapy or a combination of these. Self-help books may also be useful. It's important to remember that while depression may be a normal reaction to a diagnosis of epilepsy, this doesn't mean that it will go away by itself. The good news is that it can be successfully treated in the majority of cases.

From child to young adult – the transition

Many young people 'grow out' of epilepsy as they get older, but some types of epilepsy, such as juvenile myoclonic epilepsy, actually start during mid to late childhood and continue into adulthood. It's also possible for epilepsy to change, with seizures becoming more or less frequent, or more or less severe. If this happens it may be necessary to try a different AED, so do report any changes in the frequency, duration and severity of seizures to your specialist. In some cases, seizures will stop completely, only to return a few months or even years later.

Changes in service provision

Some types of epilepsy continue into adulthood, even if medication is controlling the seizures. This means that if medication is withdrawn, seizures start again. If your child's epilepsy continues, the management of his epilepsy will transfer from a paediatrician to a neurologist or specialist in adult epilepsy. The age at which this happens varies but is usually around 17 years old. If your child is 15 or 16 when diagnosed, he might see a neurologist straight away to avoid having to change after a year or so.

Some young people might find the change disruptive – it may be that he has to go to a different hospital, for example (although many hospitals have both child and adult services), or he may find the change of doctor upsetting. Ultimately he'll need to make the move to adult services, but if you really feel he's not ready it might be worth talking to the paediatrician about this to see if it might be helpful to arrange a joint handover (where both the paediatrician and neurologist are present). In most cases the transition is smooth, and can be a positive experience. It is a useful time for you and your child to evaluate his epilepsy care to see whether there have been any changes in the condition and whether treatment needs to be adjusted.

If at any point you're not happy with the care your child receives, whether it's through child or adult services, you can request a second opinion, or ask to be referred to a different hospital. You can find out about other hospitals and the services they offer through NHS Choices (<www.nhs.co.uk>) or Dr Foster (<www.drfoster.co.uk>). For more information, have a look at the NICE guidelines for the treatment of epilepsy in adults and children – see <www.nice.org.uk> or contact NSE or Epilepsy Action.

Becoming more independent – how will your child cope?

If your child's epilepsy continues into adulthood he'll need to start taking more responsibility for the management of his condition. As well as attending review appointments with the neurologist and being responsible for his own medication, this could mean learning how to avoid situations that may trigger a seizure, recognizing the warning signs (if he has them) that a seizure is starting and getting himself into a safe place. It may also mean learning how to talk to and explain his condition to other people.

The age at which he's ready to do this will depend on a number of factors. Young people are individuals, and your child's specific characteristics and ability will have more bearing on how capable he is of managing his epilepsy than his age – some young people are more sensible and reliable at 12 than others are at 18. You know your child best; you know his attitudes and capabilities, and this will help you to judge when he's ready to start taking more responsibility. It's a good idea to start giving him a little responsibility as soon as you think he can handle it. If he copes well with that, you can give him a little more. Tempting though it is to keep control of everything from drugs and medical appointments to where your child goes and what he does in his leisure time, if he's to have an independent life as a young adult, you'll need to trust him, and you'll need to let go.

Learning to let go – trusting your child to manage his condition

As parents it's our duty to protect our children from harm. Remember when he learned to walk? How you stood watching him, fingers crossed, silently praying he wouldn't fall and hurt himself? Of course, you took reasonable precautions – you didn't let him walk around on concrete until he mastered his balance; you didn't let him walk up and down stairs unaided until he learned to do so safely. But you stood back, and you let him take the *risk* of falling over, because that was the only way he'd learn to walk.

To an extent, you're in a similar situation when your child with epilepsy starts to grow up. You want to protect him, but wrapping him in cotton wool will only delay his ability to function independently and to have a normal, independent life. As we've seen in the previous section, the age at which a child is ready to start taking responsibility for his condition will vary, but it's up to you to start encouraging this as soon as you think the time is right – just as you did when he learned to walk. It will be natural for you to be worried about him: Will he remember to take his AEDs if I don't give them to him? He has seizures when he gets overtired – will he go to bed when he needs to if I don't nag him? He wants to go out with his friends – what if he has a seizure and I'm not there?

However, unless his epilepsy is so severe that he needs constant care, the chances are that you will have to trust him to manage these situations at some point. You will have spent a lot of time and energy discussing his condition and its management with him already; you will have explained how important it is for him to take his AEDs when he's supposed to, and avoid the situations he knows may trigger a seizure. You will have made sure that he knows what to do if he feels a seizure coming on, or that if his seizures occur without warning he is able to make a mature decision about the safety of the situations he puts himself in. Ultimately, as he moves into adulthood, it will be up to him to choose to take small risks as his social, leisure and academic or working life expands. The most important and helpful thing you can do is to keep the lines of communication open on a fairly adult and equal level; if he feels you're nagging, he's less likely to take notice of what you say, but if you advise him in a caring, non-judgemental way, he'll probably listen – even if he pretends not to!

You may feel slightly happier if you know he always has something with him that makes it clear he has epilepsy and explains how he's treated and what action, if any, should be taken if he has a seizure. There are a number of items that can be carried or worn that do this, from epilepsy ID cards (usually free from epilepsy organizations) to identity jewellery and talismans. Contact NSE or Epilepsy Action for details of how to obtain these and how they work (see Useful addresses).

9

Young people living with epilepsy 1: School, college and work

You may be a young person who's been recently diagnosed with epilepsy, or you may have been living with the condition for some years but are now becoming more independent and making more decisions about how you manage your day-to-day life. These last three chapters will hopefully provide you with lots of practical information and answer some of the questions you may have about living with epilepsy as a young person in the twenty-first century. Although earlier parts of the book have been aimed mainly at parents, you might find some of the stuff in other chapters useful, so just dip in and out as you feel like it. If you're newly diagnosed you might like to have a look at the section on reactions to diagnosis (see p. 34), and Chapter 11 touches on how you might feel about your diagnosis.

Coping with school, college and university

You may have a number of concerns about how epilepsy will affect your academic life, but the main worries will probably be:

- How your classmates and teachers will react to the knowledge that you have epilepsy.
- How they'll behave if you have a seizure.
- Whether your epilepsy will cause you to have too much time away from your studies.
- Whether you'll have a seizure in the middle of an exam.

How people react to your epilepsy depends largely on what they know about the condition; basically, the more they know about it, the less afraid they'll be and the more likely it is that it won't affect your relationship at all. It's important to remember that most people with epilepsy lead normal lives. Telling other people about the condition can help them, as well as you, to feel more at ease about it.

Depending on how severe your epilepsy is and how well your seizures are controlled, there's no reason why you shouldn't be able to achieve as much and join in (most) activities in the same way as other students. Epilepsy can make this a bit more difficult, though, so you need to be prepared for any problems and take steps to try and find solutions. In some cases, for example, epilepsy causes concentration problems, confusion, memory problems and tiredness. This may be to do with the area of your brain that's causing the epilepsy, or it may be connected with the AEDs you're taking, which can affect concentration and cause fatigue. If you're still at school, your parents will have told your teachers about your epilepsy, but if you're starting college or uni, it'll probably be down to you to tell them. If you're having trouble concentrating or keeping yourself alert during classes, it might be worth having a chat with your specialist to see if he or she thinks it could be due to side effects of your AEDs; if so, it might be possible to try a different drug or combination of drugs, or maybe to tweak the dosage. If it's the epilepsy itself that's causing the problem, discuss this with your teachers or student advisor; it may be possible for you to get some extra help. Don't be embarrassed about this – it's not your fault you're stuck with this annoying condition, and there will be plenty of other students with health problems that mean they need to do things a little differently.

What if a seizure happens during a lesson or lecture?

This is one of the reasons it's important to tell your teachers that you have epilepsy. You should tell them how often you have seizures, what form they take and how long they last. Your teachers will also need to know whether they should take any action when you have a seizure. You know how your own seizures tend to affect you, so you'll be able to give your teachers a good idea of how you're likely to feel afterwards. That way, if you need to lie down and sleep for a while, they can make arrangements for you to do this. Once you've recovered, there should be no reason why you can't return to class.

If you're at uni and find yourself attending lectures with a couple of hundred other students, there's not much point in telling that particular lecturer about your epilepsy. What might help, though, is to tell a fellow student, so that he or she knows what to do if you have a seizure during a lecture.

What about exams?

Different exam boards have different policies, as do different schools, but if you're concerned that your epilepsy may affect your performance during exams, raise this with your teachers as soon as possible so that they have time to contact the exam board if necessary. If epilepsy affects your concentration, for example, it may be possible for them to allow you extra time. If you have a seizure just before or during an exam, they may be able to take this into account when marking your paper, or they may be able to arrange a re-sit.

Bullying

Bullies tend to pick on people who they see as different in some way, and unfortunately having epilepsy could put you in this category, even though the only difference between you and anyone else is that you have a health problem to deal with. If you're unlucky enough to be bullied because of your epilepsy, try not to let it affect your confidence. If the bullies can see they're not getting to you, they're more likely to lose interest and leave you alone. If the bullying is serious or doesn't stop pretty quickly, talk about it with your parents or teachers, or telephone the helpline of one of the epilepsy charities (see Useful addresses). They should be able to advise you on what to do if you're not getting the support you need from your school. Unfortunately, because of the widespread ignorance about epilepsy, not all schools know what to do in a situation like this.

Katie is now 17 and studying happily for her A levels at sixth form college.

> College is much better than school. I started having tonic-clonics when I was in year 9, but although they said at the hospital that I probably had epilepsy, it was a while before I got the proper diagnosis. I sometimes had seizures at school, and there were a couple of girls who thought it was fun to try and wind me up. They'd keep poking me in the back or pulling my hair until I'd get so stressed I'd have a seizure. I complained to the teacher, but she said I should grow up and learn how to sort out my own disputes. The next time it happened, three of my friends came with me to the head of year and told her that I had suspected epilepsy. Because I didn't have the diagnosis, she obviously didn't believe me, and said we should all go back to class and stop this 'attention-seeking behaviour'. My friends said I should tell my mum but I knew she'd just worry all the more.
>
> Eventually I got a letter from the hospital and took it to the assistant head. They had to believe me then, but they still weren't very helpful. They did manage to stop the two girls from picking on me, but when I had a seizure they seemed to expect me to just get up afterwards and carry on with my work as though nothing had happened, when what I really needed was to sleep for a while.
>
> Now I'm at sixth form college things are much better. The teachers treat you more like an adult and when I told them I have epilepsy they didn't even ask for proof. If I have a seizure during a class, they let me go home or to the medical room to lie down. They've been brilliant, and I don't dread coming here like I used to dread going to school.

Starting work

Once you've finished your full-time education, you'll be considering what to do for the rest of your life – after a suitable post-exam relaxation break, of course! If you have epilepsy, especially if you've just been diagnosed and are still finding out about the condition, you may be worried that it will make it more difficult for you to get and keep a job. Most jobs are open to people with epilepsy, including many that were previously banned, such as the police and fire services. If someone is seizure-free whether on treatment or not, there is unlikely to be a problem unless there are specific requirements or legislation (such as for a HGV driver). When filling in a form for employment, it is best to amplify your response, for example: 'epilepsy, but seizure-free for five years'. Every applicant is now assessed on an individual basis. In the UK, people with epilepsy are protected against discrimination by the Disability Discrimination Act.

Note: The information in this section referring to restrictions, health and safety regulations, and government support and advice, applies to the UK only.

The Disability Discrimination Act (DDA)

The Disability Discrimination Act 1995 is a law that makes it illegal to discriminate against disabled people. The DDA applies to anyone who has been diagnosed with epilepsy. It means that anyone who discriminates against you because you have epilepsy is breaking the law; for example, if an employer treated you less favourably than someone else without being able to justify it. However, it's sometimes possible to justify treating someone differently because of their disability; an example might be if the treatment was to avoid risks to your safety. The DDA means employers must not discriminate unfairly in job advertisements, interviews, or when offering a job. An example would be where an employer placed unfair conditions on the job offer, such as insisting you had a driving licence even when the work is mainly office-based.

Once you actually have a job, the DDA continues to protect you to ensure that you are given the same opportunities for training and promotion as anyone else who has the necessary skills and experience. The DDA also means that employers have to make 'reasonable adjustments' to help make it possible for you to get or keep a job. This can be particularly helpful for someone with epilepsy. A reasonable adjustment might be re-arranging your working hours; for example, if you tend to have seizures in the mornings, you could start and finish work an hour or two later, so that you have time to recover and get back to normal. The Commission for Equality and Human Rights has the power to enforce the DDA, and also offers legal advice and support. Visit their website at <www.cehr.org.uk>.

Disability Employment Advisors (DEAs)

Disability Employment Advisors can help you if you're finding it hard to get a job because of your epilepsy, or if you're worried you might lose the job you already have. They can offer you lots of support and advice on looking for jobs or training, and on keeping your job. They can also carry out health assessments to help give you a clearer idea of how your epilepsy might affect the type of work or training you're able to do. They'll also have information about special schemes to help you into work or to support you at work. You can find these helpful people at your local Jobcentre or Jobcentre plus. Visit the website at <www. jobcentreplus.gov.uk>.

Restricted occupations

There are some occupations that are restricted. For example, you won't be able to join the British armed services (Army, Royal Navy, Royal Air Force) if you've been diagnosed with epilepsy. If you haven't been diagnosed with epilepsy but have had a seizure in the last four years you may also be refused entry. If you had a seizure more than four years before applying, you may be able to join the armed services but you'll be excluded from certain occupations within them.

Some jobs have restrictions because of health and safety regulations. These include jobs where you and/or members of the public might be at risk of injury if you were to have a seizure while working, for example aircraft pilot, childminder, coastguard, diver, taxi driver, police officer. If your seizures aren't controlled there are some jobs that could prove dangerous – if they involve, for example, working near open water, with high voltage or open circuit electricity, with chemicals, on isolated sites or near unguarded apparatus, machines, ovens and hotplates. The type of restriction will vary depending on the job – some jobs may require proof that you have been seizure-free for a period of time, others that you have been free of seizures from a particular age. For example, at the time of writing (2008) the Civil Aviation Authority will consider applications from those wanting to train as pilots provided they have not had a seizure since the age of five.

If you're considering a job that you think may be restricted, you'll need more detailed advice, so have a look at the employment section of the NSE or Epilepsy Action websites, or call their helplines (see Useful addresses).

Should you tell your employer you have epilepsy?

This is a tough one. Under the DDA, you don't have to tell your employer or potential employer that you have epilepsy if you don't feel it's relevant. So if, for example, your epilepsy is well controlled and it won't affect your work, you don't need to mention it unless you want to. On the other hand, if you don't mention your epilepsy on the medical questionnaire or at interview and it later becomes clear that your condition affects your ability to do the job safely and efficiently, you could be in trouble! According to the Health and Safety at Work Act (1974), employers must provide a safe workplace and protect employees from any possible danger to their health. As an employee you have a responsibility, not only for your own safety while you're at work but also that of your colleagues. So if you're applying for a job where your epilepsy could pose a risk to you, your colleagues or to the general public, you must tell the employer about your condition. If you don't, you could be dismissed for gross misconduct, although your employer would have to prove that the medical questionnaire gave you the opportunity to be specific about your condition and how it might affect the job you were applying for.

You may choose not to say anything because you don't feel it's relevant – maybe because your seizures are very infrequent or only happen at night – but if the situation changes, you can tell your employer at a later date. Your employer must then acknowledge that you're covered by the DDA (see above), which means they are obliged to make 'reasonable adjustments' to help you in your work if necessary.

If you're applying for a job, you may want to wait until the interview or until you've actually been offered the job before mentioning your epilepsy – some people just write 'discuss at interview' on the medical section of the application form. If you tell your prospective employer about your epilepsy, he or she can only ask you about it in terms of how it would affect your ability to do the job you're applying for.

Risk assessments

A risk assessment might be carried out to help establish how much of a risk your epilepsy could pose to your own and other people's safety if you were to carry out the job you want to do. Don't worry too much about this. The aim isn't to prove you're at risk and stop you from doing the job; it's to identify what risks might be involved and to look at possible ways of reducing them. So, for example, while it might be dangerous for you to work in a kitchen near a hot oven, it might be reasonably safe for you to work in areas where only cold food is prepared, such as salad or dessert preparation. Or if you did a job that occasionally required you to climb a ladder, your employer might be able to get someone else to do that part of the job, perhaps giving you extra ground-level duties to make up for it.

Obviously, the level of risk will depend on a number of factors, including the nature of the job, whether you'll be working alone or with other people, the environment you'll be working in, and the type, frequency and duration of your seizures. The person carrying out the risk assessment will also want to know how well your seizures are controlled, how long it takes you to recover from a seizure and whether you usually get a warning or aura.

It can be quite scary to start thinking about 'risk' and possible accidents, but try and remember that we all take risks every single day, whether it's running across a busy road or chopping an onion. It's impossible to avoid risk, and the fact that you have epilepsy simply means that the risks may be different, not that they're greater. In fact, when you think about it, if you know that you don't get a warning before your seizures, you're unlikely to climb a ladder to clean an upstairs window, and you'd think twice before using a chainsaw; that means you're probably less at risk of that type of accident than your parents!

Access to Work

'Access to Work' is a scheme run by Jobcentre Plus that can help you if a disability or health problem affects the way you do your job, or how you get to work. For example, it can offer financial help, towards the costs either of special equipment such as extra safety guards or of travelling to and from work. Talk to the Disability Employment Advisor at your local Jobcentre Plus about this.

Disabled Person's Railcard

If you have epilepsy you're eligible for a Disabled Person's Railcard, even if your seizures are controlled by anti-epileptic drugs. This will cost you (at the time of writing) £18 for the year, or £48 for three years, but it'll give you and an adult travelling companion a third off most standard rail fares. If you're under 16 your fares will be much cheaper anyway, but a Disabled Person's Railcard will save a third off the fare of an adult travelling with you. You can download an application form from the website at <www.disabledpersons-railcard.co.uk>. Alternatively call National Rail on 08457 48 49 50 or the Epilepsy Action helpline on 0808 800 5050.

Shift work

For some people with epilepsy feeling tired or not having a regular sleep pattern can trigger seizures. If your job involves shift work, you may have difficulty getting enough sleep, or getting regular sleep. If you become extra-tired – and people on shift work often do – you may find that your seizures increase. If this happens have a chat with your employer or line manager about perhaps changing your shift patterns or working hours. This is the sort of thing that could be regarded as a 'reasonable adjustment' under the DDA (see p. 88).

Should you tell your colleagues?

It's entirely up to you to decide whether or not you want to tell the people you work with. One thing worth bearing in mind is that if you were to have a seizure at work, colleagues who didn't know you have epilepsy might be quite shocked and frightened, whereas colleagues who know what to do because you've explained your epilepsy and seizures to them are likely to be able to help you and take care of you until you recover. Being open about your epilepsy may help your colleagues to have a more positive attitude towards the condition – it's often when people don't understand something that they're afraid of it.

10

2: Practicalities and staying safe

Having epilepsy needn't stop you taking part in most of the same sports and other leisure activities that your friends enjoy, but it's obviously best to be fully informed about what you can and can't do, and about precautions you should take to make sure you'll be safe should you have a seizure.

Driving

Note: This information applies to UK only.

If you're old enough to learn to drive, you probably can't wait to have lessons. But although having epilepsy doesn't mean you can't ever drive, there are restrictions that could delay the start of your driving life. You'll need to have been seizure-free for at least a year before you can apply for a driving licence. Or you need to have had seizures only during your sleep for at least three years. You'll still need to tell the Driver and Vehicle Licensing Authority (DVLA) or Driver and Vehicle Licensing Northern Ireland (DVLNI) about your epilepsy, and they may contact your doctor for details of your condition and treatment.

If you're already a driver when you first have a seizure, or any unexplained form of loss of consciousness, you must stop driving immediately and tell the DVLA or DVLNI – even if you haven't been diagnosed with epilepsy. There are some occasions when a seizure is classed as 'provoked', such as eclamptic seizures (which can sometimes occur in pregnancy) and seizures that happen immediately following a head injury. If you have a provoked seizure, but don't have a history of seizures, the relevant driving agency will look at your case on an individual basis. However, in most cases you should be prepared to return your licence. You could send it back with the letter, and it might be an idea to photocopy your licence and keep proof of posting. If you don't send your licence back, or if you live in Northern Ireland, they'll send you a form to complete and ask your permission to contact your doctor for a medical report. Once they receive this they'll write and tell you whether or not you can carry on driving. If not, they'll ask you to send your licence back.

It's a real pain, but if you don't tell the licensing authority and you carry on driving you'll be breaking the law and you won't be covered by insurance; and, of course, if you have a seizure while driving you'll be putting yourself and other people at risk!

If you do have to stop driving because of your epilepsy, you can apply for your licence back after you've been seizure-free for at least a year. This counts from the date you had your last seizure, not the date you send your licence back. So, for example, if you start taking anti-epileptic drugs at about the time you send your licence back, but it takes five months to get the right medicine, dosage or combination of medicines to control your seizures, it would then be around 17 months from the date you returned your licence before you could get it back. Likewise, if you want to learn to drive you can apply for a driving licence only after at least a whole year has elapsed since your last seizure.

Withdrawing from anti-epileptic drugs

If you're coming off AEDs you're at greater risk of having a seizure. The Honorary Medical Advisory Panel for neurological conditions, which advises the DVLA about epilepsy, says you shouldn't drive during the withdrawal period and for six months after the withdrawal is complete. This is advice rather than a regulation, so you don't have to tell them about this, or to return your licence, unless you live in Northern Ireland, in which case you must stop driving and inform the DVLNI whenever your medication is changed or withdrawn. They'll carry out a medical review when the change or withdrawal is complete, then let you know whether or not you can start driving again.

Sports and fitness

Lots of people with epilepsy worry that they'll be left out of all sorts of activities because of their condition, but the truth is that for many activities all you need to do is to take a few sensible safety precautions, and if necessary have someone with you who can keep you safe should you have a seizure. If your seizures are completely controlled, then you need only take the same precautions as anyone else.

In most cases, being physically active can actually help reduce the number of seizures you're likely to have, so taking part in exercise or sports is good! However, for a very small number of people with epilepsy exercise can trigger a seizure, so clearly if that applies to you you should avoid over-exertion. Similarly, taking up exercise or a sport for the first time could affect your body weight and metabolism, which could in turn make you more likely to have a seizure. It's probably a good idea to have a chat with your doctor or epilepsy nurse before taking up a new activity, especially if your seizures aren't fully controlled. Factors that could affect what activities you take part in include how often you have seizures and how severe they are, what tends to trigger them (if known), and whether you have a warning before a seizure starts.

Activities to consider

The following activities are probably safe provided you take certain precautions.

Cycling

Make sure you wear protective clothing, including a correctly fitted cycle helmet. If your seizures aren't controlled, especially if they're quite frequent or if you don't get a warning, avoid cycling on a public road, and consider cycling with someone who'd know what to do if you had a seizure.

Horse riding

Again, this could be OK as long as your seizures are well controlled, or you know that you always have a warning that gives you time to climb down from the horse. You should always wear a riding hat approved by the British Horse Society (BHS). If your seizures aren't controlled, talk to your specialist about the pros and cons of riding. It may be considered safe as long as you have someone walking alongside the horse who knows what to do if you have a seizure.

Football, rugby, hockey and other contact sports

Contact sports, with the exception of boxing, which is potentially dangerous and is probably best avoided, can usually be played safely as long as you take the normal precautions, such as wearing protective headgear as recommended by the official sporting body. If your epilepsy was caused by a head injury, your epilepsy specialist may advise against contact sports.

Racket sports

Racket sports such as tennis, badminton and squash can be very strenuous, so if you're one of those who finds that over-exertion can trigger a seizure, it's best to avoid this type of activity. It's probably a good idea to have a word with your doctor before playing this type of sport.

Climbing, abseiling, hill-walking

Anything that involves heights is potentially dangerous for someone with epilepsy (and for everyone else, come to that!). That doesn't mean it's an absolute no-no. You'll need to weigh up the risks and benefits, bearing in mind your own safety and that of other members of your party. If your seizures aren't well controlled, these might be best avoided.

Skiing

If your seizures aren't controlled it's best to avoid downhill skiing, which could clearly be dangerous. Cross-country skiing could be OK so long as you take someone with you who'd know what to do if you were to have a seizure.

Fishing

Anything near water is potentially dangerous, so never go fishing alone – and it's advisable to wear a life-jacket, just to be on the safe side.

Martial arts

It's a good idea to check with your doctor before taking part in martial arts. Make sure your instructor knows about your epilepsy and what to do if you were to have a seizure.

Swimming

Like many of the other activities mentioned here, swimming can be safe as long as you follow a few simple safety precautions. It might be worth asking for your epilepsy specialist's advice and talking over the potential risks and benefits. If you go swimming, bear in mind these safety tips:

- Don't go alone – it's best to have someone with you who'll keep an eye on you all the time, and who can help you if you have a seizure. Have a practice run-through of what your companion should do if you have a seizure while in the water. This will boost your confidence – and that of your companion!

- If there's a lifeguard or pool attendant on duty, tell him or her that you have epilepsy. If there's no lifeguard, don't swim any deeper than your companion's shoulder height.
- Avoid swimming in rivers, lakes, the sea or very cold water, all of which can be dangerous for anyone, but especially if you have epilepsy.
- Avoid swimming if you feel unwell, or if you've recently changed, withdrawn from, or missed a dose of your medication. Leave the pool if you start to feel tired, cold or unwell.
- Avoid swimming when the pool is overcrowded – if you have a seizure it might be difficult for other people to see you.
- Make sure the person going with you has read the following tips on what to do if someone has a seizure while in the water.

What to do if someone has a seizure in the water

If someone is having a tonic-clonic seizure in the water, the first sign is usually a loss of co-ordination. The swimmer's sense of direction seems vague, the swimming stroke may falter and there may be involuntary head movements. If someone has a convulsive seizure in the water, or any kind of seizure where consciousness is altered, take the following steps if possible:

- Stay in the water with the swimmer, but call for help if you need it.
- Approaching from behind, support the person's head and hold it above the surface.
- Guide her away from the sides of the pool to avoid injury.
- When possible, guide the swimmer to shallow water, keeping the head above water.
- When the jerking has stopped, try and get the swimmer on to dry land, then put her into the recovery position (see p. 23).
- Stay with her until she's fully recovered.

If you think she may have swallowed or inhaled water, or if she's suffered an injury, you may need to call an ambulance.

Safety regulations

Most sports, especially extreme sports such as hang-gliding, cave-diving and parachuting, should have a governing body that sets their safety regulations. For example, the British Sub-Aqua Club sets the regulations for scuba-diving and recommends that you should be seizure-free and off medication for five years (or three years if you have seizures only while asleep) before scuba-diving. So if you're not sure whether it would be safe to take up a particular sport (or continue with one you enjoyed before being diagnosed with epilepsy) contact the governing body for advice. The Epilepsy Action helpline (0808 800 5050) can provide contact details.

Television, computer games, cinema, and clubbing

If you have photosensitive epilepsy (PSE), where seizures can be triggered by flashing or flickering lights like the kind you often see in clubs (stroboscopic or strobe lighting), you may find that even something as everyday as watching television or playing a video game can trigger a seizure. Other triggers include using other types of computer graphics and, rarely, going to the cinema. Certain shapes and patterns may have the same effect, as can lots of different colours, sunlight coming through a line of trees or flickering on water, or the images you would see flashing past if you were to look out of the window of a fast-moving train.

If you have PSE there are some simple steps you can take to reduce the risk of a seizure:

- Watch the TV from at least two metres away and in a well-lit room.
- Don't go too close to the screen – use the remote control to switch channels.

- Turn down the brightness on a VDU or use an anti-glare screen.
- Avoid playing video games if you're tired, take frequent breaks, and play in a well-lit room to reduce flicker. Playing with a patch over one eye may also help, as PSE depends on binocular (both eyes) vision.
- If you're going to the cinema, it may be an idea to call the cinema in advance to see whether they know if the film contains sequences of flashing lights.

If you have PSE it's probably sensible to avoid situations such as nightclubs where you're likely to come across strobe lighting, but it's not always possible to know in advance. If strobe lighting does start up, cover one eye with the palm of your hand to cut down the number of brain cells stimulated by the flicker, then leave the venue. Or you could try wearing light-responsive glasses with one lens treated so that it's totally darkened. The untreated lens stays clear so you can see where you're going.

Safety at home

If your seizures aren't controlled it's sensible to take some basic safety precautions around the home to reduce your risk of injury. Obviously if you're living with your parents, in a shared house, or in university accommodation, there's a limit to changes you can make to your accommodation, but being aware of the danger areas will show you what you might be able to change or at least what it would be best to avoid.

In the kitchen

When cooking use a cooker guard if possible, and turn pan handles away from the front so that you're less likely to knock them over. Avoid heating fat or oil in a pan unless there's someone else around who could turn it off if you had a seizure. Cooking or heating stuff in a microwave is usually safer, so use that as much as possible. Don't forget that you can boil water for tea or coffee in the microwave, and because you can boil it in the cup, it saves having to lift a kettle of boiling water. Always take the plates to the pan, not the other way round.

In the bathroom

Accidents are possible whether you prefer a bath or a shower, but if your seizures are unpredictable there is a risk of drowning in the bath, so a shower is usually the best option. Sitting down in the shower will help reduce risk of injury. If you do take a bath, run the cold water first, don't have the water too deep and use a non-slip bath mat. It might be worth wrapping a folded towel around the taps and other sharp edges. Try to have someone else in the house and let them know when you're having a bath or a shower, and best to leave the door unlocked (stick an 'engaged' sign on the door). In small rooms such as kitchens, bathrooms and lavatories it's a good idea if the doors open outwards, so if you fell on the floor during a seizure someone could still get to you.

When you go to bed

If you're likely to fall out of bed, choose a low bed, or sleep on a mattress on the floor. Soft feather pillows are best avoided because of the slight risk of suffocation. Turn off electric blankets before getting into bed, and never, ever smoke in bed.

General safety around the home

Carpets are generally safer than hard floors, but make sure there are no loose stair carpets, or rugs that slip. Furniture with rounded edges or padding is obviously safer than things with sharp corners, but it's usually not realistic to change all the furniture! Just try to avoid having too much furniture in one room, and stay away from glass-topped tables! Avoid open fires, use guards for gas and electric fires and covers for radiators and hot pipes. Choose cordless electrical appliances where possible, preferably with an automatic cut-out feature. Again, it's sensible to have someone else around when you're using things like electric irons, curling tongs or hair straighteners. Make sure you have smoke alarms fitted (they're not expensive), and always replace the batteries as soon as they run low – the alarm will beep to alert you to this.

For more detailed information, Epilepsy Research has a useful free factsheet, *Epilepsy: Safety in the Home*, see <www.epilepsyresearch.co.uk>.

Seizure alert dogs

If you can't actually stop your seizures, the next best thing is to be prepared for one when it hits! This is where seizure alert dogs come in. These specially trained support dogs can tell when a seizure is about to begin. They're trained to bond very closely with their owners, so that they are completely 'in tune' with them and are therefore able to detect a change in the person long before any human could. This could be anything from a slight change in your natural scent to a change in your skin tone, or even in your eyes. The dog is trained to give a clear signal, such as circling you, pawing at the ground or barking, that a seizure is about to begin. This allows time for you to get to a place of safety until the seizure is over. This is when the dog receives a treat.

You need to be 16 or over to apply for a dog. You will need to be prepared to work very closely with the dog and its trainers in order to form the close bond and working relationship that's necessary. And obviously, you'll need to genuinely like dogs!

Things to bear in mind if you are interested in applying:

- You must have a confirmed diagnosis of epilepsy.
- You must have at least ten major seizures a month – 'major' for this purpose means tonic-clonic/atonic or complex partials, excluding sleep seizures.

- You must not undergo any changes in your medication in the six months prior to your application, nor during the training and assessment period.
- You must have a carer available, and enough daily support at home so that the dog's needs can be met at all times – he'll need his walkies and you may not always be able to take him!
- You'll need to keep accurate seizure diaries.
- Unfortunately it's not possible to train your own pet dog, and it may not be possible to place a seizure alert dog with you if you already have a dog.
- It may not be possible to train a seizure alert dog to pick up your seizures if you have a vagus nerve stimulator.

For more information about seizure alert dogs, contact the charity Support Dogs (see p. 116).

11

3: Social life and relationships

Being diagnosed with epilepsy can be quite a shock, and there are a number of things that may worry you about having the condition. For example, it can change the way you feel about yourself, and you may worry that it'll change the way other people see you, or the way your family and friends feel about you. Some people who don't know much about the condition may wrongly associate it directly with mental illness or learning difficulties – things that they also don't understand and that may scare them. This is why some people don't like to talk about the fact that they have epilepsy.

Social life

Telling your friends

Talking about any health problem can be uncomfortable, but it's only by being open about epilepsy that we can wipe out mistaken ideas about the condition and help people to understand it properly. You may decide to talk openly with your friends about your condition from the start, or you may choose to keep it to yourself until you're sure you feel confident explaining the whole thing, or you may prefer not to tell people until you have a treatment plan in place. Whatever you choose to do is a personal matter – it's your decision, and you must make it in your own time, when you've had a chance to think about it.

If your seizures happen only at night or they're well controlled with medication, you may decide you don't need to tell anyone. On the other hand, a lot of people find it helpful to discuss their condition with close friends. As we've already seen in Chapter 9, it's probably sensible to tell people about your epilepsy if you're likely to have a seizure while you're with them. You'll need to explain to your friends what might happen during a seizure and what they should do if you have one. If they know what to expect, they're less likely to be freaked out! You could use the relevant sections of this book to help you explain, or you could give them those sections to read. Alternatively, epilepsy organizations such as Epilepsy Action and the National Society for Epilepsy have plenty of booklets and factsheets you might find useful.

Going out

You might worry that epilepsy is going to affect your social life in more practical ways. For example, if you've had to give up your driving licence, getting around can be more difficult, especially if you live somewhere where public transport isn't great. Often this isn't quite such a barrier as it first seems. If you're used to driving everywhere, you probably don't even know much about the local transport system! Have a look at local bus and train timetables and try and plan your activities to fit in with these times. It probably just needs a bit of organization.

You might find you feel less confident about going out. Perhaps you're worried you may have a seizure while you're out, or maybe you're just concerned that you'll have to talk about the condition when you'd really rather not. These are perfectly normal concerns, but try not to let them affect your social life too much. Many people find that there's a period of readjustment as you get used to a slightly different way of life (such as avoiding things that may trigger seizures, and remembering to take your medication), but that things then return to near normal. You may find it helpful to talk to other young people with epilepsy, both for support and to share experiences. There are a number of online forums available where you can ask questions or just chat about epilepsy. Epilepsy Action's forum, which can be found at <www.forum4e.com>, is for those over 16 only, but the NSE has a number of forums, including one for parents, one for young people and one for the newly diagnosed. These can be found at <www.epilepsyforum.org.uk>.

Getting tired

It's important to have a social life and to take part in the same activities as your friends wherever possible, but sleep deprivation is a major trigger for many people with epilepsy, especially juvenile myoclonic epilepsy. Although it is not the 'answer', if seizures tend to be precipitated by a late night, half a clobazam tablet when you go to bed may keep you seizure-free. Consult your doctor. Otherwise, try to work out at what point your level of tiredness is likely to trigger a seizure, and just don't allow yourself to get that tired. If you know that you have a late night coming up, whether it's because you have to work a late shift or it's a social event, try to prepare by taking a brief nap in the afternoon. It also helps to try to reduce the number of other possible seizure triggers, so you might want, for example, to make sure you have regular snacks so that you don't get too hungry (see p. 60).

Alcohol

Having epilepsy doesn't mean that you can't drink at all, but it does mean that you have to be careful with drinking. Alcohol interacts with AEDs and can make them less effective, so that a seizure becomes more likely. What can also happen is that the AEDs make you more sensitive to the effects of alcohol, so you could find yourself getting drunk and/or feeling ill on a relatively small amount of alcohol. Drinking too much liquid all at once (even if it's not alcoholic) can also trigger a 'water load-induced' seizure, so stick to small quantities at a time, rather than downing two or three pints in one go.

You need to get to know how much you can drink safely. Research suggests that anything more than two units of alcohol can increase the risk of seizures, so that should be your upper limit. But that doesn't mean that two units will definitely be safe – it may be that just one unit is enough to trigger a seizure. Keeping a seizure diary (see p. 58) can help.

To give you an idea of how many units of alcohol you may be drinking you need to look at the labels. This will tell you the alcohol by volume (ABV), which is the percentage of that drink that is alcohol; if you buy a bottle of wine that has '12% alcohol by volume' on the label, it means that 12 per cent of the wine is pure alcohol. When you know the ABV, you can work out how many units you're drinking. Simply multiply the number of millilitres by the ABV, then divide that figure by 1,000. The answer is the number of units in the drink. For example:

Half a pint (284 ml) of 4% ABV beer: 284 × 4 = 1,136 ÷ 1,000 = 1.1 unit

One 175ml glass of 12% ABV wine: 175 × 12 = 2,100 ÷ 1,000 = 2.1 units

Pub measure (25ml) of spirits (40% ABV): 25 × 40 = 1,000 ÷ 1,000 = 1 unit

Never be pressurized into drinking more than you want to, and don't forget about low-alcohol beers and wines, as well as soft drinks, fruit juices and good old plain, cheap tap water! As blood levels drop overnight and the next day after a 'binge', this alone can precipitate seizures, sometimes in people without epilepsy.

Recreational drugs

There is some evidence that 'street' drugs, such as marijuana or cannabis, ecstasy, amphetamines (speed), solvents, cocaine and heroin can trigger seizures. Cocaine and heroin can trigger seizures even in people with no history of epilepsy. Taking drugs can also cause you to miss meals, forget to take your medication or not get enough sleep, all of which can lead to more seizures. Ecstasy contains chemicals that can overstimulate the nervous system, leading to seizures. Also, if you take ecstasy to help keep you dancing all night, you can become dehydrated as a result of all the physical exercise. This means you're likely to drink a lot of water over a short period of time, leading to too much fluid in the body, which can also cause a seizure. If you have epilepsy it really is best to stay off the drugs!

Smoking

Although there is currently no evidence to suggest that smoking cigarettes or cigars can trigger seizures, some nicotine preparations – such as the patches or chewing gum some people use to help them give up smoking – may, very rarely, cause convulsions. If you're trying to quit smoking (and if you do smoke you really should be trying to quit!) talk to your doctor or epilepsy specialist about the most appropriate methods of giving up.

Relationships

Boyfriends and girlfriends

Meeting someone with whom you would like to have an intimate relationship can be scary for anyone – male or female, young or old, with or without epilepsy. It's as though we're suddenly seeing ourselves as others might see us: Am I good-looking enough/clever enough/funny enough for this person to be interested in me? Do I come from the right part of town? Do I listen to the right music? That person's reaction to everything we do or say becomes vital, and this can make you reluctant to tell him or her about your epilepsy, even if you've been happily discussing the condition with your other friends for ages. It's quite natural to worry about this – you might equally worry how that person might react to your love of football or your obsession with *Star Wars*, or the fact that your dad's a lawyer or a cleaner, or that you live in a tiny apartment or a huge house. Do you see my point? It's the fact that you want to seem perfect to that person that's causing the worry – what you *think* will be perfect in his or her eyes, that is.

In fact, that person is probably worrying just as much about what you think of him or her. That doesn't mean that talking about your epilepsy will necessarily be easy, but nor does it mean that it'll be any more difficult than talking to your other friends. Your condition is part of who you are. As least, it is right now. If you don't discuss it with your partner early in your relationship, you'll spend ages worrying about when to bring it up. Many people find it a relief to confide in their partners, who often become the greatest source of support.

Sex and contraception

OK, so you've told the object of your desire about your epilepsy, and there's no dimming of love's eternal flame. Your relationship deepens, one thing leads to another and ...

You're gripped with panic again. Will your epilepsy affect your chosen method of contraception? What if having sex triggers a seizure? Again, these are normal worries, shared by many people with epilepsy. In fact, you're no more likely to have a seizure during sex than at any other time, so just be aware of possible triggers, such as tiredness, in the same way you normally would, and discuss this with your partner.

When it comes to choosing an appropriate method of contraception, there are some things you may need to take into consideration.

The pill

Oral contraceptive pills, both the combined oestrogen and progesterone pill, which are widely used, and the less common progesterone-only or 'mini pill', can be affected by some anti-epileptic drugs. This is because some AEDs speed up the way in which the liver breaks down the pill, making it less effective in preventing pregnancy. Discuss this with your epilepsy specialist. It may be possible to change to a different AED that won't affect the pill. Alternatively, your doctor may suggest another form of contraception.

Contraceptive patch

These release oestrogen and progesterone into the blood, instead of these hormones being swallowed in pill form. There is not enough information on whether this is a suitable method of contraception for women with epilepsy, but there are likely to be problems with many of the commonly used AEDs.

Contraceptive injections

Depo-Provera injections don't interact with AEDs, so these can be used if you have epilepsy.

Barrier methods (condoms, diaphragms)

There could be problems with using these if your epilepsy causes you to have periods of memory loss or confusion. However, it may be possible to overcome these by discussing the situation with your partner, who could help make sure that the condom or diaphragm is properly in place before you start having sex.

Intrauterine device (IUD)

Also called the 'coil', the IUD is a small device that is fitted into the uterus. IUDs are not affected by anti-epilepsy drugs, but there is a very small risk that you might have a reflex seizure as the device is being fitted. It's best to tell the person fitting the device that you have epilepsy, just in case this should happen.

Intrauterine system (IUS)

Similar to the IUD, this is a small device that is fitted into the uterus, but unlike IUDs the IUS contains the hormone progesterone. However, because it is released directly into the uterus rather than travelling around the body, it is not affected by anti-epilepsy drugs. Like the IUD there is a very small risk that you might faint as the device is being fitted, but this is rare.

Emergency contraception (the 'morning after' pill)

This is an emergency method of preventing pregnancy which can be used if you've had unprotected sex, or if you suspect your contraception may have failed. You can take this if you have epilepsy, but if you're taking certain AEDs you'll need a larger dose, and this needs to be prescribed by a doctor because it can't be bought from a pharmacy in the same way that the normal dose can. Try to see a doctor as soon as you know you need emergency contraception.

The best thing to do is to have a chat with your doctor about the various contraceptive options when you think your relationship is likely to become a sexual one.

Planning a family

If you're already in a life partnership and thinking of starting a family, you may be worried about how your epilepsy might affect this. Many women with epilepsy have perfectly normal pregnancies, but there is a slightly increased risk of complications. If you're planning a family it's a good idea to seek preconception counselling before you start trying for a baby. This will be an opportunity to discuss the possible effects your epilepsy and AEDs may have on your pregnancy, and to find out if changes can be made to your treatment to reduce the risk of any problems.

If you have epilepsy you're at slightly increased risk of having a baby with minor congenital abnormalities, such as small fingers and toes with small nails, club foot and facial abnormalities. There's also a slight risk of what are known as major

congenital malformations (MCMs). These could include malformations of the spinal cord (spina bifida), heart, ribs, bladder,
sexual organs, and the fingers and toes (such as unseparated
fingers). To give you a rough idea of the element of risk, any
woman in the general population has around a 1–2 per cent
risk of having a baby with an MCM; in a woman with epilepsy
who's not taking AEDs the risk is about 3.5 per cent, and slightly
higher than that in women taking one AED; and in a woman
taking two or more AEDs the risk is increased to approximately
6 per cent. These are very rough figures because there are other
factors involved, including the type of AED you take and the
size of the dose.

The risk of AEDs causing a malformation is greatest during
the first three months, as that is when the organs are formed,
so if at all possible seek preconception counselling. If you find
you're pregnant before having counselling, don't stop taking
your AEDs as this could increase the frequency of your seizures,
which could cause more problems than the AEDs themselves.
Make an appointment to see your doctor as soon as you know
you're pregnant.

Pregnancy

For many women pregnancy doesn't seem to affect the frequency of their seizures, but around 10–30 per cent of women
will have more seizures while pregnant. Some women will have
fewer seizures than before they were pregnant. Pregnancy can
cause the levels of AEDs in your blood to fluctuate, which can
affect the number of seizures you have; it's important that you
are monitored closely while pregnant so that the dosage of your
AEDs can be adjusted if necessary. It's unlikely that your baby
will be harmed during a seizure, but it's possible, so the aim is to
keep you as seizure-free as possible during your pregnancy.

Many women fear that they will have a seizure while giving
birth, but according to research published in 2006 in the journal

Neurology, this happened in only around 3.5 per cent of the cases studied, and these were more likely where the woman had had a previous seizure during pregnancy. You'll probably be advised to have your baby in hospital, so that doctors and midwives can make sure you're properly cared for during labour and delivery. Make sure you take your AEDs with you and that you take them at the right time. There are a number of pain relief options that are suitable for women with epilepsy, including epidural anaesthetic, as long as the anaesthetist is aware that you have epilepsy and knows what medication you're taking. Gas and air is fine, but be careful not to over-breathe while using it as this can trigger seizures in some people.

For more information on pregnancy, birth and coping with a new baby when you have epilepsy, contact one of the epilepsy organizations such as NSE or Epilepsy Action.

Conclusion

There is no doubt that having epilepsy changes your life, even if it's only to the extent that you have to take medication every day. If you're a young person with epilepsy (or the parent of one) here are a few reasons to think positively about the future:

- Depending on the type of epilepsy, it's not uncommon for seizures to just stop of their own accord.
- There is a great deal you can do to reduce the risk of seizures, for example by identifying and avoiding triggers, and by making sure you take your medication exactly as prescribed – yes, it's a pain, but it's a small price to pay for a relatively seizure-free existence.
- Research into epilepsy continues apace, and with each passing year doctors understand more about the condition, enabling them to develop new effective drug and surgical treatments. This means that the outlook for people with epilepsy is better than ever before.
- Although the stigma surrounding epilepsy still presents one of the biggest challenges for people with the condition, things are improving. With more media attention, more well-known people speaking out and wider forms of communication such as the internet, there is now an increasing level of awareness and knowledge among the wider public.

The vast majority of people with epilepsy lead very normal and ordinary lives. Others lead lives that can only be described as extraordinary, achieving great things in the worlds of sport, media, music, theatre, art, literature and politics. Alfred Nobel, the man who invented dynamite and founded the Nobel Prize, was thought to have had epilepsy; so was the Russian writer Dostoevsky, the military general Napoleon and the philosopher

Socrates. More recent examples of famous people with epilepsy include Rabbi Lionel Blue, actor and director Danny Glover, singer/songwriter Neil Young and comedian Rik Mayall. Of course, you don't have to be famous to lead a full, productive and enjoyable life. Epilepsy will undoubtedly affect your life, but it doesn't have to ruin it!

Useful addresses

Benefit Enquiry Line
Tel.: 0800 882 200
Website: www.dwp.gov.uk

The Government has set up another
website (www.direct.gov.uk/en/
DisabledPeople/index.htm) to help
disabled people access more information
and services. See also **Jobcentre Plus.**

The Brain Injury Association (see
Headway)

**British Complementary Medicine
Association**
PO Box 5122
Bournemouth BH5 0WG
Tel.: 0845 345 5977
Website: www.bcma.co.uk

Cerebra
Second Floor Offices
The Lyric Building
King Street
Carmarthen SA31 1BD
Tel.: 01267 244 200
Website: www.cerebra.org.uk

Provides information and support for
brain-injured children and young people
and their parents and carers.

Citizens Advice (operating name of the
**National Association of Citizens Advice
Bureaux)**
Tel.: 020 7833 2101
Website: www.citizensadvice.org.uk

Contact A Family
209–211 City Road
London EC1V 1JN
Helpline: 0808 808 3555
Website: www.cafamily.org.uk

Gives details of UK support groups for
parents and carers of children with certain
syndromes.

Disability Alliance
Universal House
89–94 Wentworth Street
London E1 7SA
Tel.: 020 7247 8776 (administration only)
Website: www.disabilityalliance.org

**Driver and Vehicle Licensing Agency
(DVLA)**
Drivers Customer Services (DCS)
Correspondence Team
DVLA
Swansea SA6 7JL
Tel.: 0870 240 0009
Website: www.dvla.gov.uk

**Driver and Vehicle Licensing Northern
Ireland**
Driver Licensing Division
County Hall
Castlerock Road
Coleraine
Co. Londonderry BT51 3TB
Tel.: 0845 402 4000
Website: www.dvlni.gov.uk

Epilepsy Action
New Anstey House
Gate Way Drive
Leeds LS19 7XY
Tel.: 0113 210 8800
Helpline: 0808 800 5050
Website: www.epilepsy.org.uk

Epilepsy Bereaved
PO Box 112
Wantage
Oxon OX12 8XT
Tel.: 01235 772850
Website: www.sudep.org

Epilepsy Scotland
48 Govan Road
Glasgow G51 1JL
Tel.: 0141 427 4911
Helpline: 0808 800 2 200
Website: www.epilepsyscotland.org.uk

Epilepsy Wales
Bradbury House
22 Salisbury Road
Wrexham LL13 7AS
Helpline: 08457 413774
Website: www.epilepsy-wales.org.uk

FABLE (For a Better Life with Epilepsy)
Lower Ground Floor
305 Glossop Road
Sheffield S10 2HL
Tel.: 0114 275 5335
Freephone Advice Line: 0800 521 629
Website: www.fable.org.uk

Gamma Knife Centre
Cromwell Hospital
Cromwell Road
London SW5 0TU
Tel.: 020 7460 2000
Website: www.gammaknife.co.uk

Gamma Knife surgery enables patients
to undergo a non-invasive form of
neurosurgery and can be an alternative to
open surgery.

Headway (the Brain Injury Association)
7 King Edward Court
King Edward Street
Nottingham NG1 1EW
Tel.: 0115 924 0800
Helpline: 0808 800 2244
Website: www.headway.org.uk

**Institute for Complementary and
Natural Medicine**
Can-Mezzanine
32–36 Loman Street
London SE1 0EH
Tel.: 020 7922 7980
Website: www.icnm.org.uk

International Bureau for Epilepsy
11 Priory Hall
Stillorgan
Dublin 18
Ireland
Tel.: 00 353 1 210 8850
Website: www.ibe-epilepsy.org

Jobcentre Plus
Tel.: 0845 6060 234 (seeking work); 0800
055 6688 (seeking benefit claim)
Website: www.jobcentreplus.gov.uk

Part of the Department of Work and
Pensions; gives details of local offices and
telephone numbers.

London Gamma Knife Centre
154 Harley Street
London W1N 1HH
Tel.: 020 7486 6969
Website: www.radiosurgery.co.uk

**National Bureau for Students with
Disabilities (see Skill)**

**National Institute for Health and
Clinical Excellence (NICE)**
71 High Holborn
London WC1V 6NA
Tel.: 0845 003 7780
Website: www.nice.org.uk

National Society for Epilepsy (NSE)
Chesham Lane
Chalfont St Peter
Bucks SL9 0RJ
Tel.: 01494 601300
UK Epilepsy Helpline: 01494 601400 (10
a.m. to 4 p.m., Monday to Friday)
Website: www.epilepsynse.org.uk

**Royal Society for the Prevention of
Accidents (RoSPA)**
RoSPA House
Edgbaston Park
353 Bristol Road
Birmingham B5 7ST
Tel.: 0121 248 2000
Website: www.rospa.co.uk

**Skill: National Bureau for Students with
Disabilities**
Chapter House
18–29 Crucifix Lane
London SE1 3JW
Tel.: 020 7450 0620 (also textphone)
Information service: 0800 328 5050;
textphone 0800 068 2422
Website: www.skill.org.uk

The Society of Homeopaths
11 Brookfield
Duncan Close
Moulton Park
Northampton NN3 6WL
Tel.: 0845 450 6611
Website: www.homeopathy-soh.org.uk

Support Dogs
21 Jessops Riverside
Brightside Lane
Sheffield S9 2RX
Tel.: 0114 261 7800
Website: www.support-dogs.org.uk

Further reading

Andermann, Lisa, *Epilepsy in Our World: Stories of Living with Seizures from Around the World*, Oxford University Press USA, 2007.

Appleton, Richard, *The Illustrated Junior Encyclopaedia of Epilepsy*, Petroc Press, 1995.

Appleton, Richard, Brian Chappell and Margaret Beirne, *Epilepsy and Your Child*, 2nd edition, Class Health, 2004.

Appleton, Richard and Tony Baldwin (eds), *Management of Brain Injured Children*, 2nd edition, Oxford University Press, 2006.

Brodie, Martin, *Fast Facts: Epilepsy*, 3rd edition, Health Press, 2005.

Buchanan, Neil, *Understanding Epilepsy: What it is and How it Can Affect your Life*, Simon and Schuster, 2003.

Freeman, John, Eric Kossoff, Jennifer Freeman and Millicent Kelly, *The Ketogenic Diet: A Treatment for Children and Others with Epilepsy*, 4th edition, Demos, 2007.

Freeman, John, Eileen Vining and Diana Pillas, *Seizures and Epilepsy in Childhood: A Guide for Parents*, Johns Hopkins University Press, 2003.

Gay, Kathlyn and Sean McGarrahan, *Epilepsy: The Ultimate Teen Guide*, Scarecrow Press, 2007.

Gumnit, Robert, *Your Child and Epilepsy: A Guide to Living Well*, Demos, 2005.

Kutscher, Martin, *Children with Seizures: A Guide for Parents, Teachers and Other Professionals*, Jessica Kingsley, 2006.

Marshall, Fiona and Dr Pamela Crawford, *Coping with Epilepsy*, new edition, Sheldon Press, 2006.

Singh, Anuradha, *100 Questions and Answers About Your Child's Epilepsy*, Jones and Bartlett, 2008.

In addition, there are a number of excellent books, DVDs and videos available from the epilepsy organizations NSE and Epilepsy Action.

Index

117